RICHARD H. HAUG, DDS, CONSULTING EDITOR

ATLAS OF THE ORAL AND MAXILLOFACIAL SURGERY CLINICS OF NORTH AMERICA

Multidimensional Diagnosis and Treatment Planning in Maxillofacial Surgery

MARIA J. TROULIS, DDS, MSc, GUEST EDITOR

VOLUME 13 • NUMBER 1 • MARCH 2005

W.B. SAUNDERS COMPANY
A Division of Elsevier Inc.
PHILADELPHIA LONDON TORONTO MONTREAL SYDNEY TOKYO

W.B. SAUNDERS COMPANY
A Division of Elsevier Inc.

The Curtis Center • Independence Square West • Philadelphia, Pennsylvania 19106
http://www.oralmaxsurgeryatlas.theclinics.com

ATLAS OF THE ORAL AND MAXILLOFACIAL SURGERY CLINICS OF NORTH AMERICA
March 2005
Editor: John Vassallo

Volume 13, Number 1
ISSN 1061-3315
ISBN 1-4160-2823-4

Atlas of the Oral and Maxillofacial Surgery Clinics of North America (ISSN 1061-3315) is published biannually by W.B. Saunders Company. Corporate and editorial offices: The Curtis Center, Independence Square West, Philadelphia, PA 19106-3399. Accounting and circulation offices: 6277 Sea Harbor Drive, Orlando, FL 32887-4800. Subscription prices are $145.00 for US subscribers, $169.00 for US nonsubscribers, $184.00 for international subscribers, $220.00 for international non-subscribers. Single issue price is $110.00. Foreign air speed delivery is included in all *Clinics* subscription prices. All prices are subject to change without notice. POSTMASTER: Send address changes to *Atlas of the Oral and Maxillofacial Surgery Clinics of North America*, W.B. Saunders Company, Periodicals Fulfillment, Orlando, FL 32887-1800. **Customer Service: 1-800-654-2452 (US). From outside of the US, call 1-407-345-4000. E-mail: hhspcs@wbsaunders.com.**

Atlas of the Oral and Maxillofacial Surgery Clinics of North America is covered in Index Medicus.

Printed in the United States of America.

CONSULTING EDITOR

RICHARD H. HAUG, DDS, Professor of Oral and Maxillofacial Surgery; and Associate Dean for Clinical Affairs, Division of Oral and Maxillofacial Surgery, University of Kentucky College of Dentistry, Lexington, Kentucky

GUEST EDITOR

MARIA J. TROULIS, DDS, MSc, Department of Oral & Maxillofacial Surgery, Massachusetts General Hospital, Boston, Massachusetts

CONTRIBUTORS

ARNULF BAUMANN, MD, DMD, Associate Professor, University Hospital of Cranio-Maxillofacial and Oral Surgery, Medical University of Vienna, Vienna, Austria

NINA BROGLE, MD, Neuroradiology Fellow, Department of Radiology, Massachusetts General Hospital, Boston, Massachusetts

PAUL CARUSO, MD, Assistant in Radiology, Department of Radiology, Massachusetts Eye and Ear Infirmary, Boston, Massachusetts; Assistant in Radiology, Massachusetts General Hospital, Boston, Massachusetts; and Instructor in Radiology, Harvard Medical School, Boston, Massachusetts

HUGH D. CURTIN MD, Professor of Radiology, Harvard Medical School, Boston, Massachusetts; and Chief of Radiology, Department of Radiology, Massachusetts Eye and Ear Infirmary, Boston, Massachusetts

THOMAS B. DODSON, DMD, MPH, Director of Resident Training, Department of Oral and Maxillofacial Surgery, Massachusetts General Hospital; and Associate Professor, Department of Oral and Maxillofacial Surgery, Harvard School of Dental Medicine, Boston, Massachusetts

ROLF EWERS, MD, DMD, Professor and Chairman of University Hospital of Cranio-Maxillofacial and Oral Surgery, Medical University of Vienna, Vienna, Austria

JAIME GATENO, DDS, MD, Associate Professor, Department of Oral and Maxillofacial Surgery, Dental Branch, The University of Texas Houston Health Science Center, Houston, Texas

LEONARD B. KABAN, DMD, MD, W.C. Guralnick Professor and Chairman, Department of Oral and Maxillofacial Surgery, Massachusetts General Hospital, Boston, Massachusetts

DAVID A. KEITH, BDS, FDSRCS, DMD, Professor, Department of Oral and Maxillofacial Surgery, Massachusetts General Hospital; Harvard School of Dental Medicine, Boston, Massachusetts

RON KIKINIS, MD, Associate Professor, Radiology; Director, Harvard Surgical Planning Laboratory, Brigham and Women's Hospital, Boston, Massachusetts

CLEMENS KLUG, MD, Resident, University Hospital of Cranio-Maxillofacial and Oral Surgery, Medical University of Vienna, Vienna, Austria

MARY JANE O'NEILL, MD, Instructor in Radiology; Director, Ultrasound Services, Division of Abdominal Imaging and Interventional Radiology, Massachusetts General Hospital, Boston, Massachusetts

KURT SCHICHO, DSc, Scientist, University Hospital of Cranio-Maxillofacial and Oral Surgery, Medical University of Vienna, Vienna, Austria

EDWARD B. SELDIN, DMD, MD, Associate Professor of Oral and Maxillofacial Surgery, Massachusetts General Hospital, Boston, Massachusetts

JOHN F. TEICHGRAEBER, MD, FACS, Professor, Division of Pediatric Surgery, Department of Surgery, Medical School, The University of Texas Houston Health Science Center, Houston, Texas

PETRA THURMÜLLER, MD, DMD, Resident in Oral and Maxillofacial Surgery, Knappschaftskrankenhaus Bochum-Langendreer, Universitätsklinik, Schornau, Bochum, Germany

ARNE WAGNER, MD, DMD, Associate Professor, University Hospital of Cranio-Maxillofacial and Oral Surgery, Medical University of Vienna, Vienna, Austria

JAMES J. XIA, MD, PhD, Assistant Professor, Department of Oral and Maxillofacial Surgery, Dental Branch; and Assistant Professor, Division of Pediatric Surgery, Department of Surgery, Medical School, The University of Texas Houston Health Science Center, Houston, Texas

KRISHNA C. YESHWANT, BS, Student, Harvard Medical School, Boston, Massachusetts

CONTENTS

FORTHCOMING ISSUES

September 2005

Bone Grafting
George M. Kushner, DMD, MD, *Guest Editor*

March 2006

Implant Procedures
Michael S. Block, DMD, *Guest Editor*

PREVIOUS ISSUES

September 2004

Maxillofacial Cosmetic Surgery, Part II
John E. Griffin, Jr, DMD, *Guest Editor*

March 2004

Maxillofacial Cosmetic Surgery, Part I
John E. Griffin, Jr, DMD, *Guest Editor*

September 2003

Endoscopic Techniques in Oral and Maxillofacial Surgery
Larry L. Cunningham, Jr, DDS, MD, *Guest Editor*

ELSEVIER
SAUNDERS

Atlas Oral Maxillofacial Surg Clin N Am 13 (2005) vii–viii

Atlas of the
Oral and
Maxillofacial
Surgery Clinics

Preface

Multidimensional Diagnosis and Treatment Planning in Maxillofacial Surgery

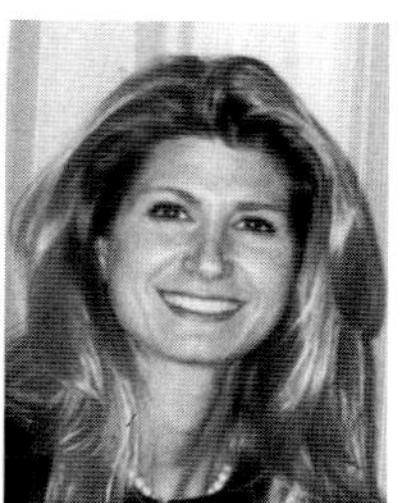

Maria J. Troulis, DDS, MSc
Guest Editor

> We are now at the point where we must educate people (surgeons) in what nobody knew yesterday, and prepare in our schools (training programs) for what no one knows yet but what some people must know tomorrow. —Margaret Mead

Minimally invasive surgery is defined as "the discipline of surgical innovation combined with modern technologies" [1]. It is only during the past 10 years that oral/maxillofacial surgeons have become interested in altering our "maximally invasive" procedures with the use of novel minimally invasive techniques.

At the Massachusetts General Hospital, our initial interest in minimally invasive surgery was driven by our research and clinical work in distraction osteogenesis. This interest quickly broadened to include the development of "totally buried, remotely activated miniature devices" to be placed through minimally invasive endoscopic approaches. The realization that totally buried devices did not allow for midcourse corrections led us to pursue the development of three-dimensional (3-D) treatment planning imaging and software. Our group envisions a day when patients requiring maxillofacial reconstruction will have detailed 3-D computed tomographic images, a treatment plan developed with 3-D virtual modeling, skeletal expansion through endoscopically placed miniature totally buried distraction devices remotely or continuously activated, and, when necessary, tissue-engineered grafts.

Currently, the range of new technologies developing in our specialty includes new imaging modalities and applications, surgical navigation, and advanced treatment planning and modeling. These are aspects of evolving technologies and are the subject of this issue of the *Atlas of the Oral and Maxillofacial Surgery Clinics of North America*. Advances are not limited to these areas, however, and the future is without limits. It is with great excitement that I pursue research and the clinical use of advanced technologies with my mentor, Leonard B. Kaban, and our entire Massachusetts General Hospital team.

I hope that this issue, which is dedicated to diagnosis and treatment planning using advanced technologies, stimulates interest in novel treatments for our patients. I want to take this opportunity to thank the contributing authors for their enthusiasm, their expertise, and their

1061-3315/05/$ - see front matter
doi:10.1016/j.cxom.2004.12.004

commitment to minimally invasive surgery and imaging. I am sure you as the reader will agree that these articles are exciting and of high quality.

Maria J. Troulis, DDS, MSc
Department of Oral & Maxillofacial Surgery
Massachusetts General Hospital
55 Fruit Street
Boston, MA 02114-2692, USA

E-mail address: mtroulis@partners.org

Reference

[1] Hunter JG, Sackier JM. Minimally invasive high tech surgery: into the 21st century. In: Hunter JG, Sackier JM, editors. Minimally invasive surgery. Columbus: McGraw-Hill, Inc.; 1993. p. 3–6.

ELSEVIER
SAUNDERS

Atlas Oral Maxillofacial Surg Clin N Am 13 (2005) 1–12

Atlas of the Oral and Maxillofacial Surgery Clinics

A Computer-Assisted Approach to Planning Multidimensional Distraction Osteogenesis

Krishna C. Yeshwant, BS[a,*], Edward B. Seldin, DMD, MD[b], Ron Kikinis, MD[c], Leonard B. Kaban, DMD, MD[b]

[a]*Harvard Medical School, Boston, MA*
[b]*Department of Oral and Maxillofacial Surgery, Massachusetts General Hospital, 32 Fruit Street, Boston, MA 02114, USA*
[c]*Harvard Surgical Planning Laboratory, Brigham and Women's Hospital, 75 Francis Street, Boston, MA 02115*

The introduction of CT and MRI into the clinical environment has dramatically improved the diagnosis of and treatment planning for craniofacial anomalies. These imaging technologies in combination with sophisticated image processing software and powerful graphics hardware have enabled surgeons to model patient anatomy and plan procedures with unprecedented speed and accuracy. The digital reconstruction of two-dimensional (2D) CT slices into a 3D CT model (Fig. 1), for instance, has become a particularly valuable technique in assessing craniomaxillofacial anomalies.

The 3D CT image relates the positions of several distant anatomic features (eg, the orbita, zygoma, maxilla, and mandible), which allows surgeons to more readily appreciate a patient's skeletal deformity as a three-dimensional whole (sagittal, coronal, and horizontal planes) rather than as a series of two-dimensional CT slices. This three-dimensional approach to diagnosis and treatment planning is important because most congenital and acquired facial deformities involve one or more planes and may be asymmetric.

There are currently two distinct approaches to three-dimensional craniofacial treatment planning. In the first approach, an operation is performed on customized 3D acrylic models of the skull that are produced using CT data and stereolithography. Although this technique allows surgeons to use familiar surgical tools to simulate a procedure, the process is time consuming and expensive. Furthermore, the quantitative analysis of the planned movements or comparison of different plans is not possible. To address these limitations, software has been developed by Everett et al for interactive surgical simulation of craniomaxillofacial reconstructive procedures using 3D CT data.

In this article we describe the use of a CT-based 3D treatment planning software package to analyze craniomaxillofacial deformities. The software allows the surgeon to determine the parameters of movement of the proposed correction and to prescribe the radius of curvature and the placement of a specific semiburied curvilinear distraction device to accomplish the proposed correction and to evaluate the outcome.

Protocol

The CT-based treatment planning software package (3D Slicer) described in this article (Fig. 2) was developed as a research project through the Surgical Planning Laboratory at Brigham and Women's Hospital (Boston, MA) in collaboration with the General Electric Corporate Research and Development Center (Schenectady, New York) and the media

* Corresponding author.
E-mail address: Krishna_yeshwant@hms.harvard.edu (K.C. Yeshwant).

1061-3315/05/$ - see front matter
doi:10.1016/j.cxom.2004.10.001

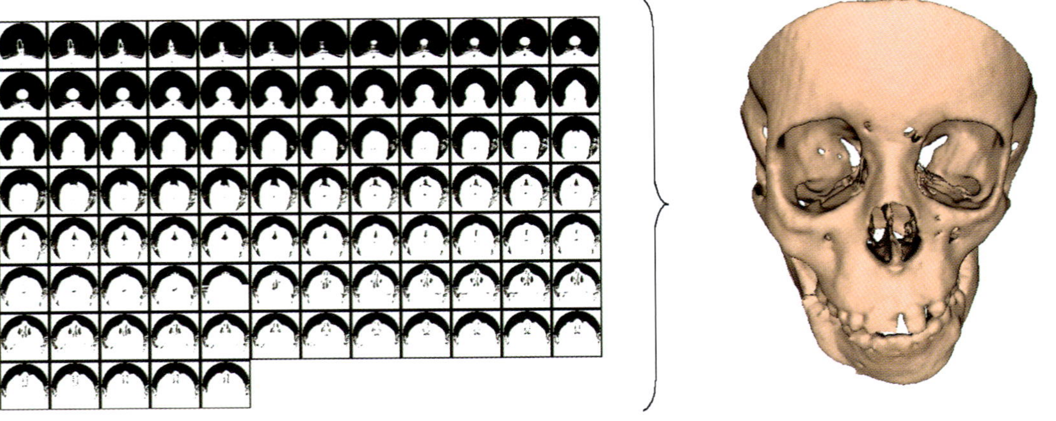

Two-Dimensional CT Scan Slices

Three-Dimensional CT Reconstruction (3D CT)

Fig. 1. 3D CT models are reconstructed from multiple two-dimensional CT slices. The 3D CT scan in this figure was reconstructed using the marching cubes algorithm.

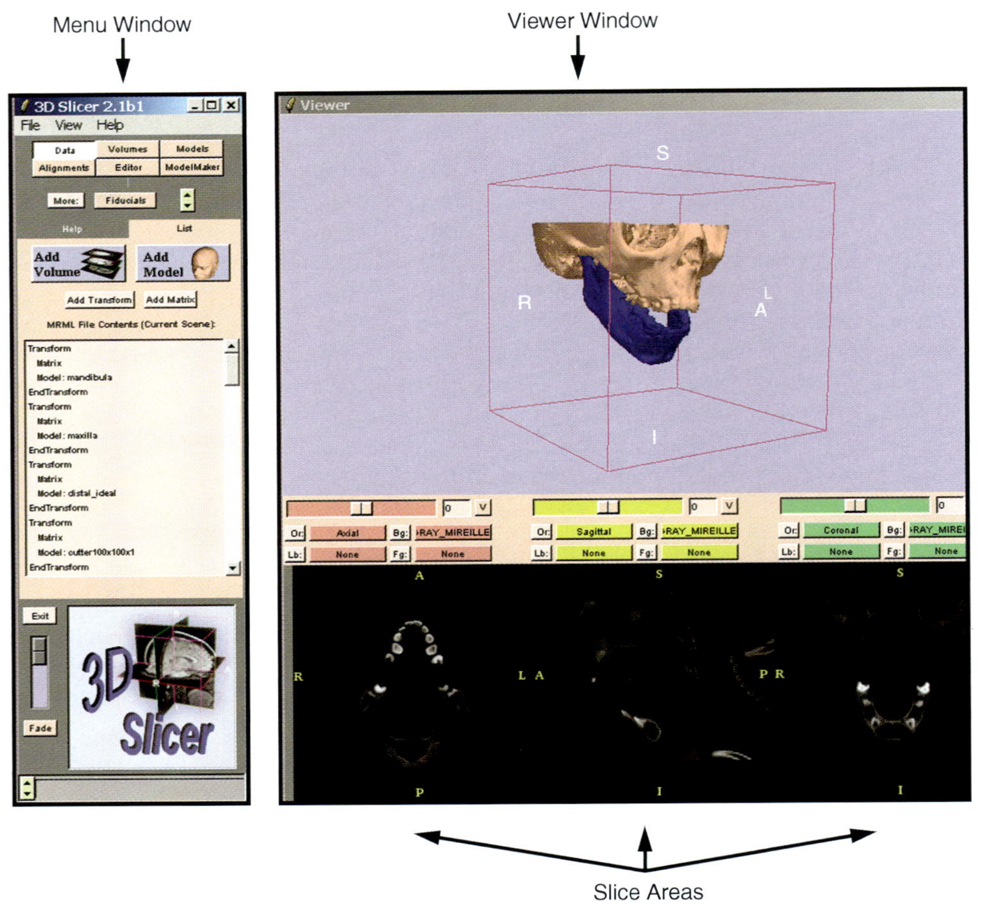

Fig. 2. The 3D Slicer is an open-source medical visualization application that can be downloaded through the World Wide Web at www.slicer.org. The narrow window on the *left* is called the "Menu" window and contains all the major user interface elements for image manipulation, model reconstruction, and treatment planning. The window on the *right* is called the "Viewer" window and contains a main viewing area that is used to display 3D models. The *bottom quarter* of the Viewer window can be used to show three slice areas (*arrows*) that are used to display a 2D multiplanar reformatted version of the imported volume. User commands issued in the menu window are visualized in the Viewer window.

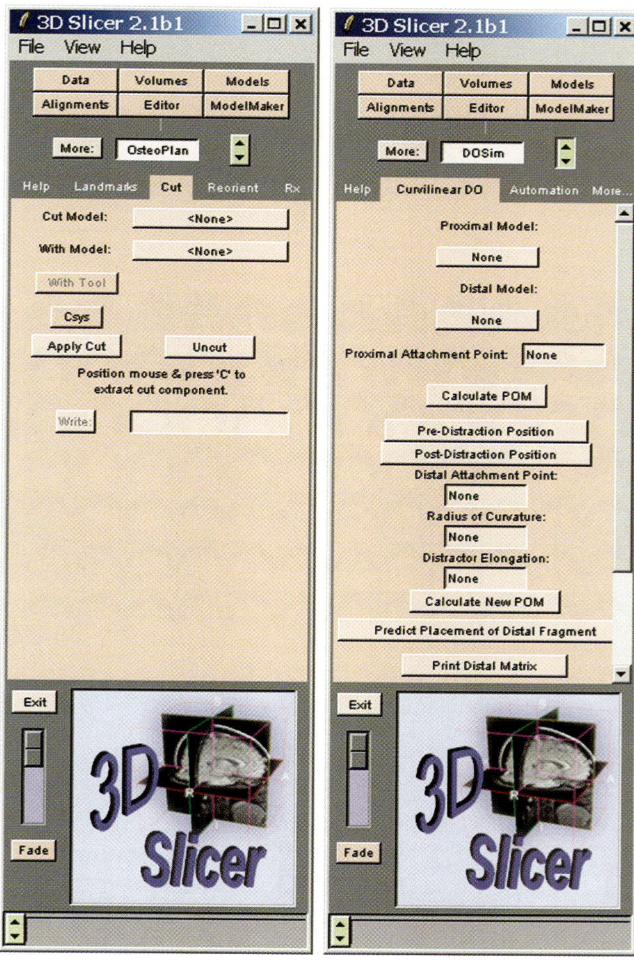

Fig. 3. The OsteoPlan module (*left*) and the DOSim module (*right*) are accessed through the "More" dropdown menu located in the menu window. The OsteoPlan module is used to simulate osteotomies, and the DOSim module is used to calculate curvilinear prescriptions.

laboratory of the Massachusetts Institute of Technology (Cambridge, MA). It is an open-source visualization application that runs on multiple operating systems and hardware configurations including UNIX-based workstations, Linux workstations, and Windows (Microsoft, Seattle, Washington) operating system. The techniques describe in this article were executed on Solaris-based workstations (Sun Microsystems, Santa Clara, California) with a Windows operating system. The application and source code for the 3D Slicer are freely available through the World Wide Web at www.slicer.org. The craniofacial customizations discussed throughout this article are contained in the OsteoPlan and DOSim (Surgical Planning Laboratory, Brigham and Women's Hospital, Boston, Massachusetts and the Oral and Maxillofacial Surgery Department, Massachusetts General Hospital, Boston, Massachusetts) (Fig. 3) modules of the 3D Slicer.

Data acquisition

Axial and coronal CT scans of the patient's facial skeleton are acquired with no intervening gaps at a 1.25-mm slice thickness with a 512 × 512 pixel matrix using standard head and neck scanner settings. The patient is asked to wear a bite splint during the scan to separate the upper and lower teeth to facilitate the segmentation process described below. For young patients, the CT scans must be taken as close to the time of operation as possible to minimize planning errors caused by patient growth.

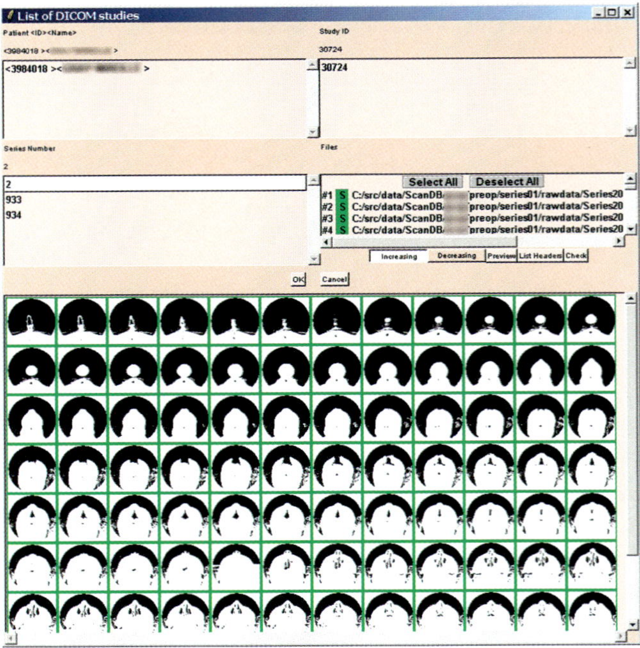

Fig. 4. The DICOM reader built into the 3D Slicer automatically identifies the header information from the selected CT data on the clinician's computer. When the user clicks "OK," the CT data will be loaded into the 3D Slicer.

Image processing

After image acquisition, the patient's CT data are transferred from the console of the scanner to the clinician's computer (using SUN, Linux, or Windows operating systems) over an Ethernet network. The CT data are loaded into the 3D Slicer and examined for scanning errors. The 3D Slicer can read several types of medical image volumes, including Signa and Genesis data (General Electric, Schenectady, New York), and digital imaging and communications in medicine (DICOM) slices. The authors' group most commonly uses DICOM images from Lightspeed (General Electric) or SOMATOM Sensation 16 (Siemens, Munich, Germany) scanners. These images are loaded into the 3D Slicer through a DICOM reader (Fig. 4).

One of the CT scans is selected for use in treatment planning. The selected scan data are filtered using a "Window/Level" feature that allows the user to emphasize the borders of the facial skeleton without obscuring the scan images (Fig. 5).

The software is then used to identify bony anatomic structures from the CT scan in a process known as segmentation. The purpose of this process is to separate the maxilla from the mandible to facilitate later treatment planning steps. During segmentation, the user labels the mandible with one color and the skull base with another in each slice of the CT scan (Fig. 6). This labeling process can be completed in approximately 15 minutes if a bite splint is used during the CT scan, using semiautomated image processing-based algorithms (analogous to the "fill tool" used in photographic editing software). However, if a splint is not used, segmentation may require more than 1 hour of manual effort.

The segmentation data are fed into an algorithm that reconstructs 3D surface models (3D CT scans) of the patient's mandible and skull base (Fig. 7). Two-dimensional images of the 3D models can be displayed on the computer monitor or printed.

Treatment planning

The reconstructed models are placed in a standardized starting position by identifying three landmarks (the menton, the nasion, and the anterior nasal spine) on the mid-sagittal plane of the reconstructed models. In addition, the right and left orbitale are identified on the horizontal plane of the models. The treatment planning software aligns these landmarks and the associated skeletal models to the true vertical and horizontal planes using a least squares method algorithm.

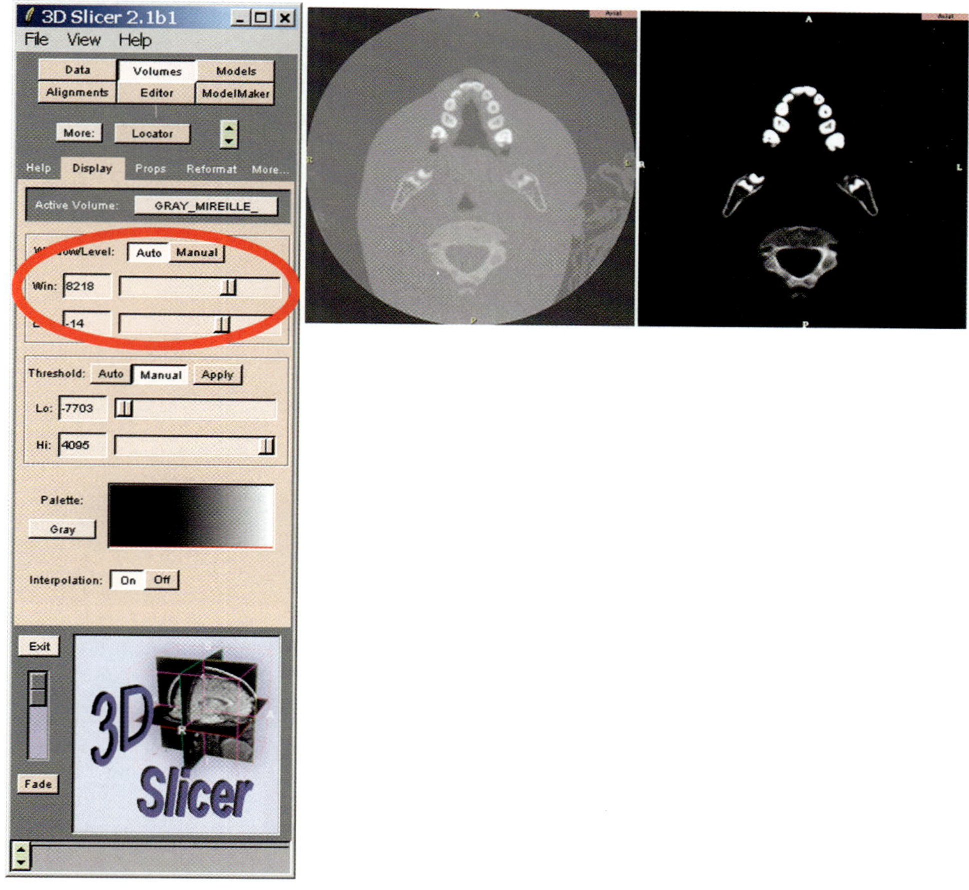

Fig. 5. The Window/Level feature allows the user to set the pixel values that will have the most visible range of color values. This allows the user to emphasize entities in the scan that have a similar density. In the authors' studies, skeletal structures are emphasized. The user interface for this feature is *circled* in the menu window. One of the original axial slices from a patient CT scan is shown in the *middle*. The same axial slice is shown (*right*) after the color values were adjusted to emphasize the skeletal features.

Landmarks are then used to quantitatively assess the patient's deformity by calculating relative facial proportions. Craniofacial surgeons review the 3D reconstructions in the laboratory along with the patient's measurements, photographs, radiographic images, and other clinical data to formulate surgical strategies. The treatment planning software is used simulate the outcomes of these strategies.

To simulate the corticotomies required in distraction osteogenesis, a cutting tool is positioned with respect to the mandible using a movable coordinate system (Fig. 8). The desired corticotomy generally extends from the junction of the ramus and body of the mandible at the upper border to the angle of the mandible at the lower border. Once the desired corticotomy position is identified with the cutting tool, the cut operation is applied, and two topologically closed models are created (Fig. 9). This operation is repeated on the opposing side of the mandible in cases involving bilateral surgery. The resultant models are then repositioned using the movable coordinate system (Fig. 10). The treatment planning software checks for bony interference ("collision") as the models are moved. In some cases, a virtual coronoidectomy is required to position the bone fragments ideally (Fig. 11). Multiple treatment plans may be developed for each patient. These plans can be superimposed on the preoperative models to illustrate the prescribed movement (Fig. 12). The surgeon then chooses a final treatment plan.

Once the ideal bone positions have been determined, the treatment planning system is used to calculate the curvilinear path of motion required for each skeletal correction (both sides in bilateral cases). Each curvilinear movement is based on an axis of rotation about which the mandibular movement occurs (Fig. 13). The surgeon then uses landmarks to identify regions on

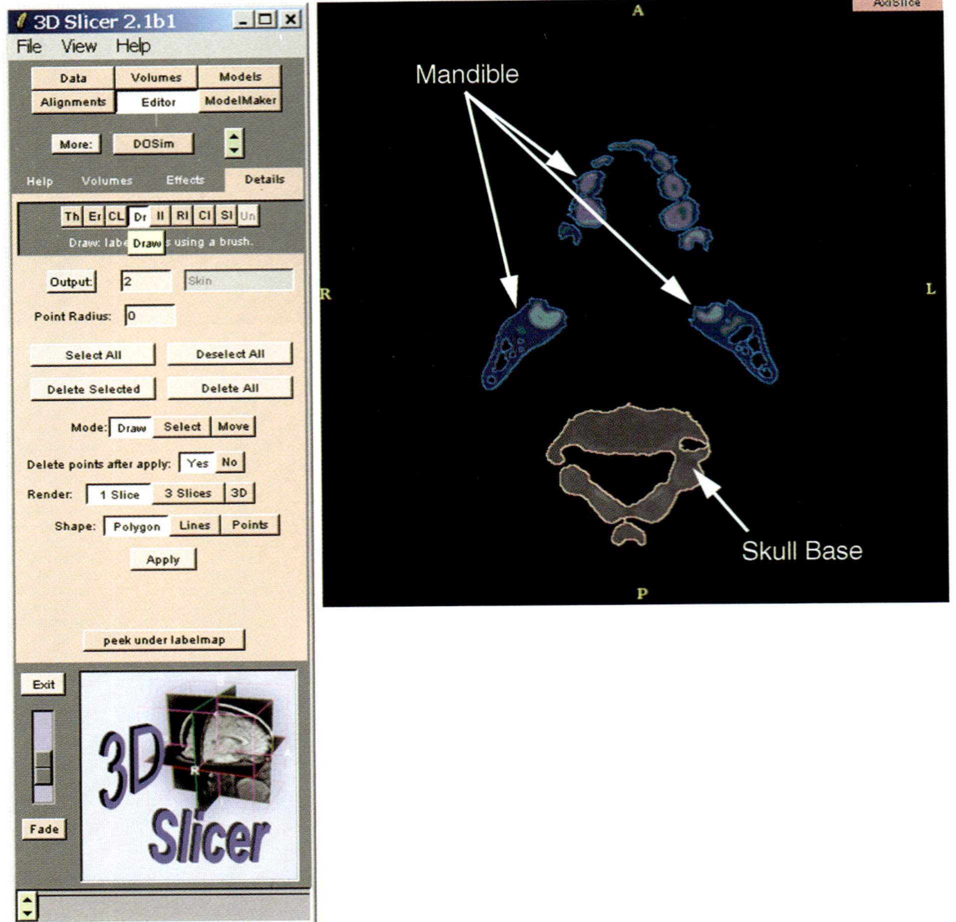

Fig. 6. During segmentation, the user uses the "Editor" module (*left*) to create label maps in which a unique label is assigned to each tissue type. The Editor module was used to label the mandible and the skull base in the image shown (*right*) (each entity is labeled with a different color). If a bite splint is not used, the user must manually identify skeletal structures by outlining their borders in several of the CT slices.

the patient's mandible that encompass acceptable attachment points for the footplates of the distraction devices. The treatment planning system is then used to automatically prescribe one device from a kit of five curvilinear distractors and to indicate the ideal placement of that device.

Transfer to the operating room

A model of the prescribed curvilinear distractor is obtained from the manufacturer and overlaid on the patient's mandible model (Fig. 14). The footplates of the distractor model are used to locate the positions of the drill holes that need to be made in the patient's mandible to attach the curvilinear device. Landmarks are placed on the mandible model at these positions. The 3D coordinates of the landmarks can be used as targets within an intraoperative 3D navigation system that would guide the surgeon's drill bit to the correct location on the patient's mandible in the operating room (Fig. 15). This approach is ideal because it allows screws to be placed without direct visualization of the mandible, thus enabling an intraoral approach.

Alternatively, a customized drill guide can be made (based on the patient's 3D model) that is intraoperatively overlaid on the mandible to identify the location of the required drill holes. This technique requires an extraoral approach to provide enough space to place the drill guide. Currently, the surgeon places the device based on multiple two-dimensional printouts produced from the 3D treatment planning model.

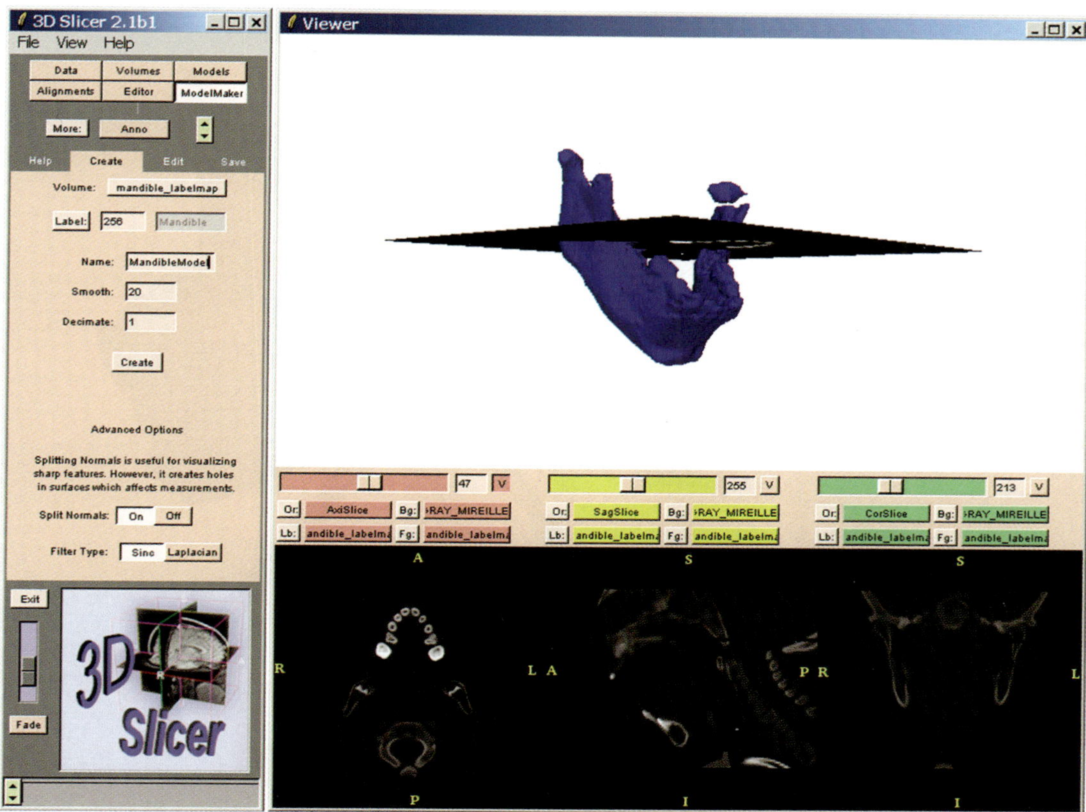

Fig. 7. The 3D Slicer uses the marching cubes algorithm to reconstruct a 3D surface model based on a series of 2D CT scans. The interface to this algorithm is exposed through the ModelMaker module as shown in the Menu window (*left*). In the example shown here, a series of segmented images named "mandible_labelmap" are used to create a mandible model named "MandibleModel." The reconstructed mandible model is shown in the Viewer window on the right.

Surgical technique

Before surgery, frontal, lateral, and oblique images of the patient's 3D treatment plan are prepared. An incision is made to expose the angle and ramus of the mandible. Two footplates of the device are removed from the curvilinear distractor in the operating room (Fig. 16). With the mandible exposed, the corticotomy is marked, and the curvilinear distractor is oriented on the angle based on the treatment plan images. Using a sterile lead pencil, the locations of the drill holes are marked. The device is removed, and the corticotomy is made through the buccal and lingual cortices using a reciprocating surgical saw. The curvilinear distractor is fixed with two screws on both the anterior and posterior footplates. The device is activated to provide tension across the wound, and the corticotomy is completed using an osteotome. The device is then turned back and elongated to 1 mm. The wound is copiously irrigated with saline and closed in layers. Postoperative radiographs, photographs, and CT scans are taken. The distraction protocol consists of day 0 latency and a rate of 0.5 mm, twice per day, for as many days as necessary to achieve the desired elongation.

Summary

Although 3D treatment planning offers several advantages in preparing for craniofacial procedures, there are still several problems to be solved. First, the lack of accurate dentition in 3D CT scans limits the use of 3D treatment planning techniques to relatively severe cases in which attaining optimal occlusion is not the primary objective. In addition, the lack of

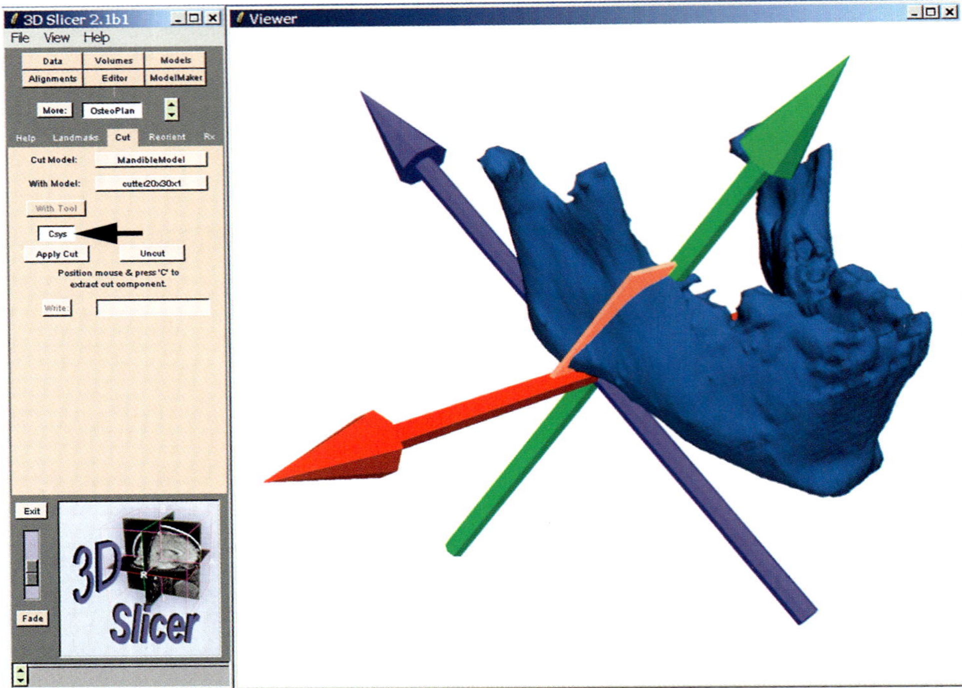

Fig. 8. The movable coordinate system is displayed or hidden by pressing the Csys button (*arrow*) in the OsteoPlan module. The movable coordinate system can be attached to any model loaded into 3D Slicer. In this example, the coordinate system is attached to the rectangular cutting tool. By clicking and dragging on the coordinate system (ie, *large arrows* in the Viewer window), the user can translate and rotate the attached model. This figure illustrates how the cutting tool is positioned with respect to the mandible at the desired corticotomy location. Note that the Viewer window can be reconfigured to show only the 3D view.

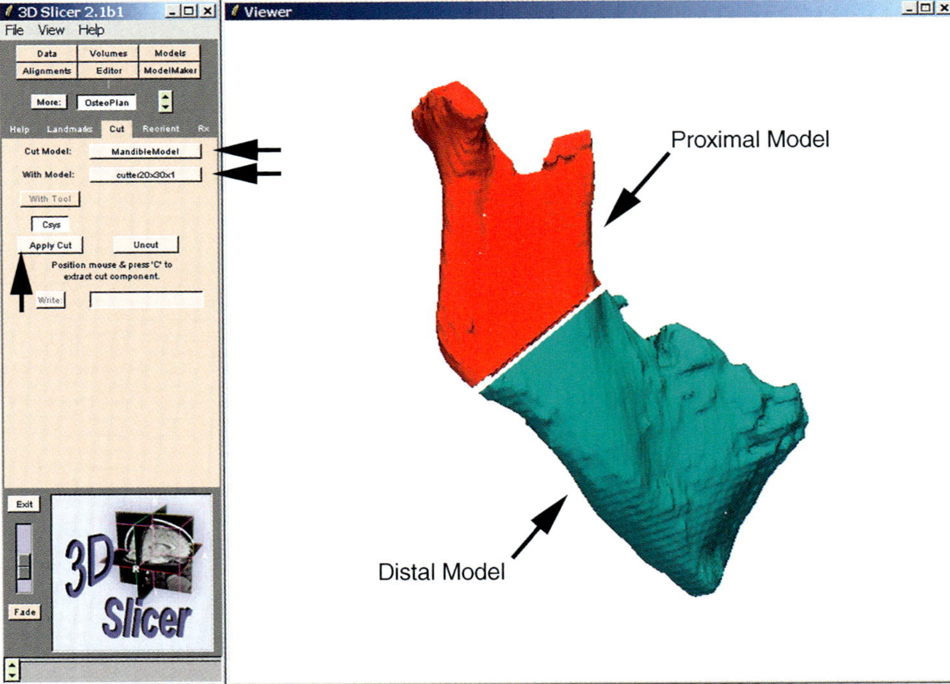

Fig. 9. The cut operation is applied when the user selects the "Cut Model" and the "With Model" (*left arrows*) in the OsteoPlan module and clicks on the "Apply Cut" button (*left arrow*). In this figure, the user cut the mandible model using the cutter model, resulting in two topologically closed models, the proximal and distal models (*right arrows*).

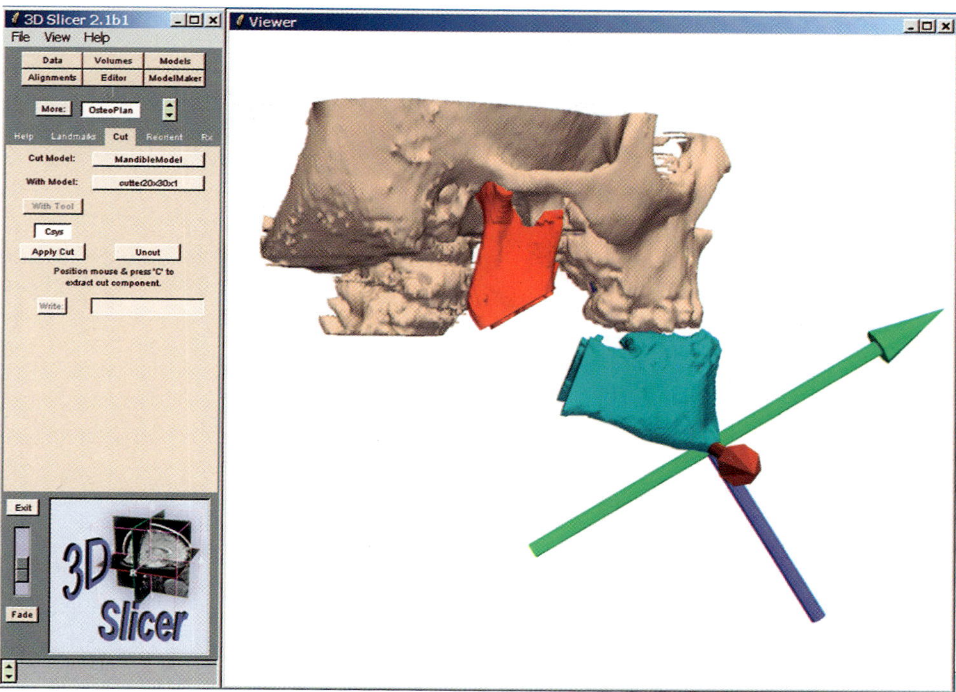

Fig. 10. The resultant cut models are repositioned into their ideal positions using the movable coordinate system by attaching the models to the coordinate system and moving the coordinate system. In this example, the distal fragment is repositioned with respect to the maxilla (*large arrow*).

well-established 3D cephalometrics limits the ability of the system to quantify and track skeletal changes. Furthermore, the time and computer expertise currently required to produce a treatment plan is a significant barrier for most surgeons. The lack of a fourth dimension in treatment planning, that is, the dimension of growth over time, also limits the applicability of the system, as does the limitation of the system in the representation of soft tissue contours. Finally, navigation systems to facilitate the intraoperative implementation of treatment plans are essential to fully realize the benefits of a three-dimensional treatment planning system.

Continuing efforts in the development of the authors' three-dimensional treatment planning system have been directed at addressing these issues. The use of high-resolution volumetric CT scanning technologies, laser scans of a patient's dental models, and improved reconstruction

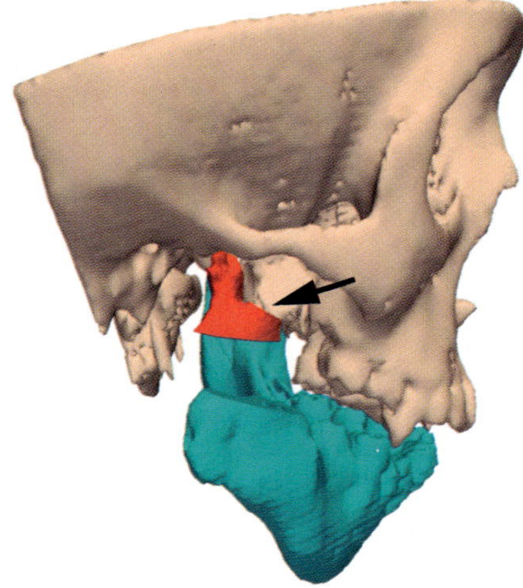

Fig. 11. Coronoidectomies are performed when bony interference (*arrow*) is predicted by the treatment planning system.

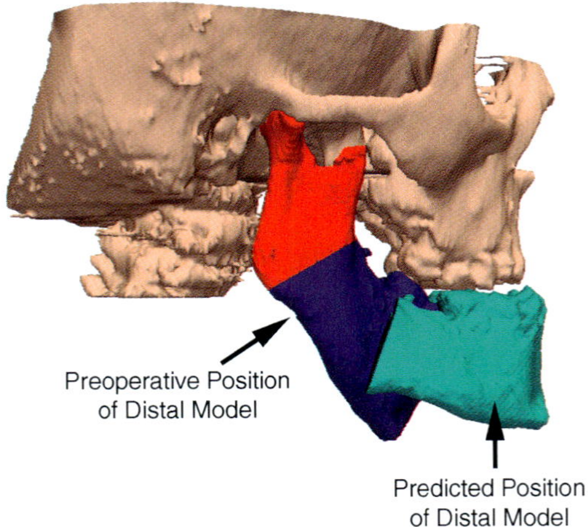

Fig. 12. Treatment plans can be superimposed on the preoperative models to illustrate the prescribed movement.

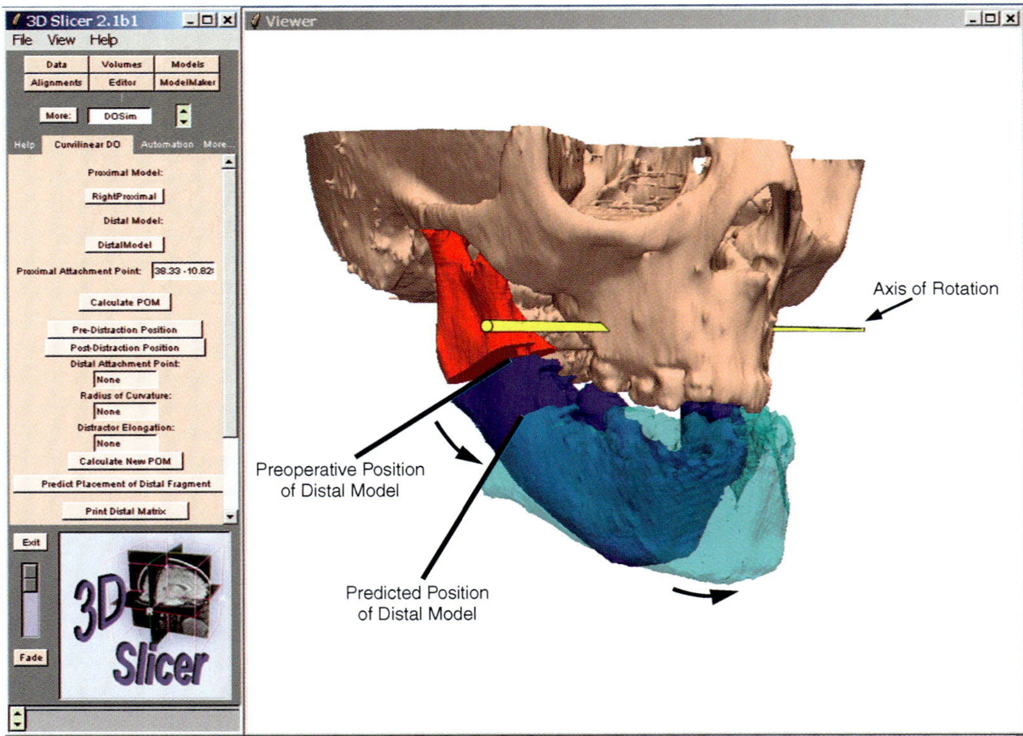

Fig. 13. The *line* running through the maxilla in this image represents the axis of rotation (*right arrow*) around which the preoperative distal model must rotate to be placed in the predicted position. The *curved arrows* represent the curvilinear movement of the distal model as it moves into the predicted position. The axis of rotation is used along with radius of curvature, pitch, and handedness parameters to prescribe a specific curvilinear device. Note that any model loaded in the treatment planning system can be made transparent, as is done here with the distal model.

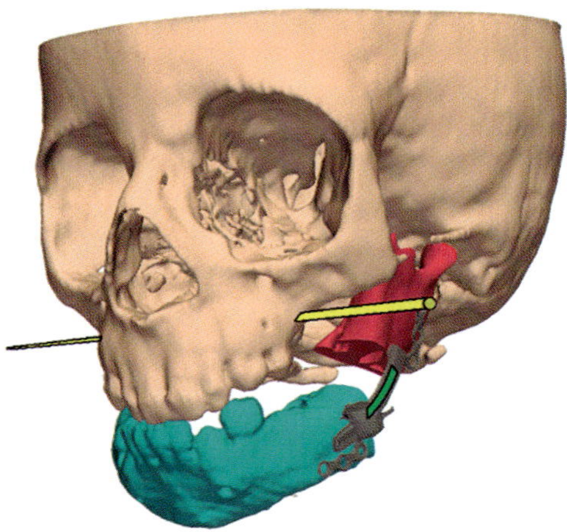

Fig. 14. A fully planned procedure with overlaid and cut distractors.

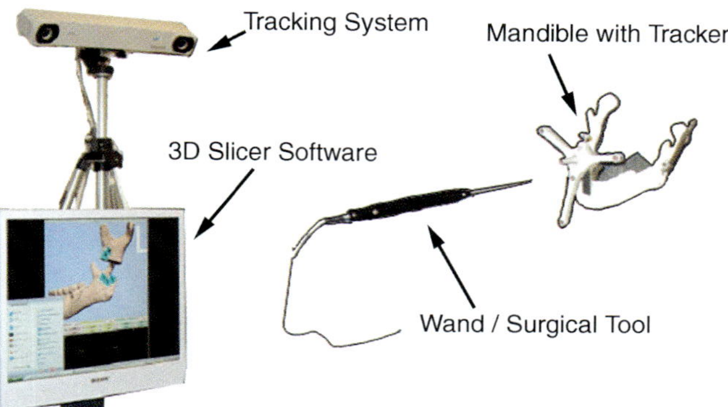

Fig. 15. In this surgical navigation system (Courtesy of R. Ellis, PhD), a wand is used to locate drill holes on the mandible by registering the location of the wand in the operating room with the 3D plan developed in the 3D Slicer. As the surgeon moves the wand, the tracking system indicates where the tip of the wand is located in 3D Slicer. In this way, drill holes can be placed to within 0.5 mm of the desired location.

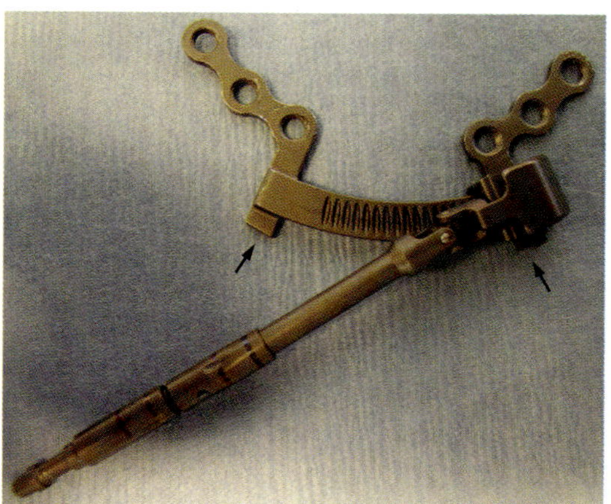

Fig. 16. Two footplates are removed (*arrows*) from the curvilinear distraction device in the operating room to reduce the size of the device.

methods will be used to address the lack of accurate dental data. A study is underway to establish 3D cephalometrics. Simplified user interfaces will help to streamline the planning process to ease the learning barrier for surgeons. Efforts also are being directed at integrating CT-guided navigation systems for intraoperative navigation.

Although significant resources are still required to successfully use the tools described in this article, the benefits offered by 3D treatment planning can be great. As the limitations discussed earlier are addressed and as the cost of high performance graphics hardware and navigation instrumentation continues to drop, access to these tools will increase, and the use of 3D reconstructions will eclipse the current use of 2D images as the standard for planning complex craniofacial surgeries.

Further readings

Altobelli DE, Kikinis R, Mulliken JB, et al. Computer-assisted three-dimensional planning in craniofacial surgery. Plast Reconstr Surg 1993;92:576–85 [discussion 586–7].

Everett PC, Seldin EB, Troulis MJ, et al. A 3-D system for planning and simulating minimally-invasive distraction osteogenesis of the facial skeleton. Presented at the 3rd International Conference on Medical Image Computing and Computer-Assisted Intervention. Pittsburgh, Pennsylvania, October 11–14, 2000.

Marsh J, Vannier M. Comprehensive care for craniofacial deformities. St. Louis: Mosby. 1985.

Marsh J, Vannier M, Stevens WG, et al. Computerized imaging for soft tissue and osseous reconstruction in the head and neck. Clin Plast Surg 1985;12:279–91.

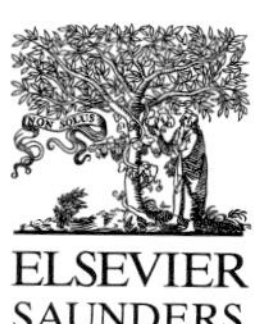

ELSEVIER
SAUNDERS

Atlas Oral Maxillofacial Surg Clin N Am 13 (2005) 13–23

Atlas of the
Oral and
Maxillofacial
Surgery Clinics

Geometric Considerations in the Transition from Two-Dimensional to Three-Dimensional Treatment Planning

Krishna C. Yeshwant, BS[a], Petra Thurmüller, MD, DMD[b], Edward B. Seldin, DMD, MD[c,*]

[a]*Harvard Medical School, Boston, MA*
[b]*Knappschafts Krankenhaus Bochum-Langendreer, Universitätsklinik, Schornau, Bochum, Germany*
[c]*Department of Oral and Maxillofacial Surgery, Massachusetts General Hospital, 32 Fruit Street, Boston, MA 02114, USA*

Scratch the surface of daily existence and a remarkable complexity is immediately revealed. In this article we set the goal of presenting a common sense explanation of some of the geometry that lies below the surface of orthognathic treatment planning. An appreciation of how objects move in space—starting with two dimensions and moving to three dimensions—is helpful in understanding some of the complexities of treatment planning as presented in several other articles in this issue.

Orthodontists and surgeons who are engaged in treatment planning use cephalometric norms for angular and linear measurements. In planning a correction, these measurements are usually considered and manipulated separately. Most clinicians recognize that objects that move freely in space have six "degrees of freedom": **rotational movements**, known as yaw, pitch, and roll, plus **translational movements** along three orthogonal axes. Less generally appreciated, but fundamental to a full understanding of treatment planning, is the fact that ***combinations of translational and rotational movements of a solid object in three-dimensional space from an initial to a final position can be resolved into a net movement that follows a helical path about a specific axis***. If the pitch of the helix happens to be zero, the motion is a simple rotation about the axis. If the pitch is infinite, then the motion is a pure translation parallel to the axis.

A nonmathematician's explanation, starting with basic considerations in plane geometry

Before examining objects in three-dimensional space, let us start with an inventory of the ways in which two lines can relate to each other in two-dimensional space. In Euclidean, two-dimensional space, two lines either **intersect** or are **parallel**; there are no other alternatives (Fig. 1). This small but exhaustive menu of options has important consequences for how objects move in two dimensions.

Let us consider the net movement of an object in two-dimensional space (eg, the tracing of a mandible from a cephalometric radiograph) from an initial to a final position. We represent this movement as the change in the coordinates of two arbitrary landmarks (points A and B) connected by a line segment (A-B), which moves with the object to A'-B' (Fig. 2). The extended lines of which these two segments are parts either intersect or are parallel to each other. Line segments that connect A to A' and B to B' describe the net movement of each of the paired landmarks (Fig. 3).

* Corresponding author.
E-mail address: seldin.edward@mgh.harvard.edu (E.B. Seldin).

1061-3315/05/$ - see front matter
doi:10.1016/j.cxom.2004.12.002

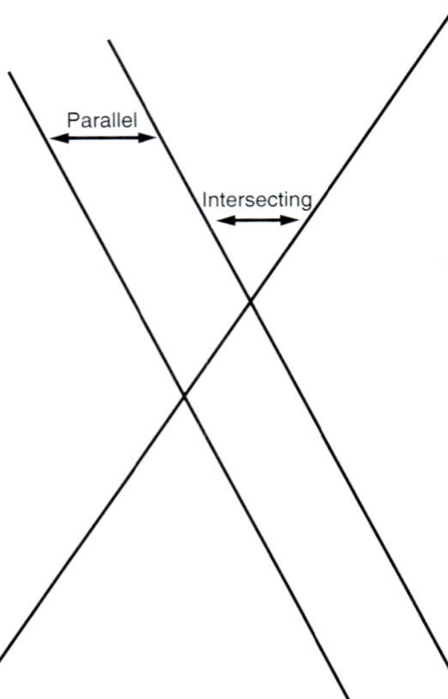

Fig. 1. In two-dimensional space, lines either **intersect** or are **parallel**. There are no other alternatives.

Using a straight edge and a compass, let us construct the perpendicular bisectors of lines A-A' and B-B' (Fig. 4). It is an axiom of plane geometry that these bisectors also must intersect or be parallel to each other. If they intersect, they do so at a point that is the center of a circle or concentric circles, of which lines A-A' and B-B' happen to be chords (Fig. 5). (Euclid is credited with the observation that perpendicular bisectors of such chords intersect at the center of the circle). No matter how circuitous the path taken by the object in moving from A-B to A'-B', the simplest description of the net movement is to say that the object followed an ***arcuate path*** of a specific length (or angular displacement) about the center point identified previously (Fig. 6). If, however, the line segments A-A' and B-B' happen to be parallel, then their perpendicular bisectors also must be parallel. In this unique circumstance, one might say that the "center of rotation" for a purely translational movement is at infinity.

Three-dimensional space

In three-dimensional space, rotation of objects occurs not around a central point, as it does in two dimensions, but about an ***axis***. An axis is a line that has a specifiable ***orientation in space*** and traverses any plane it intersects at a specifiable point. In two-dimensional space, a given line segment has only one perpendicular bisector. In three-dimensional space, however, an infinity of

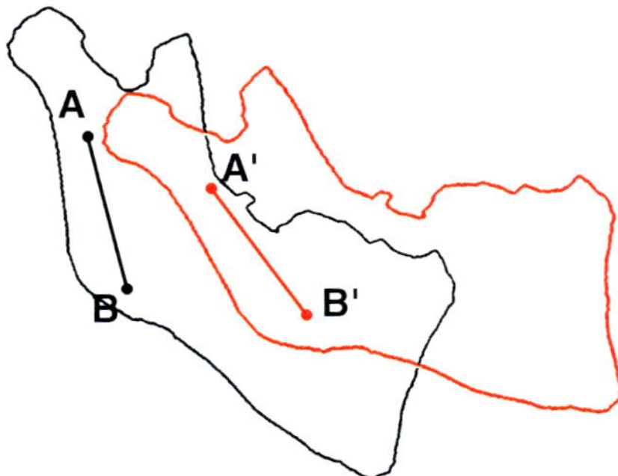

Fig. 2. A tracing of a mandible moved from one position to another in two dimensions. The black tracing is the initial position and is represented by landmarks. A and B are connected by a line segment, A-B. A'-B' represents the final position of the tracing, in red.

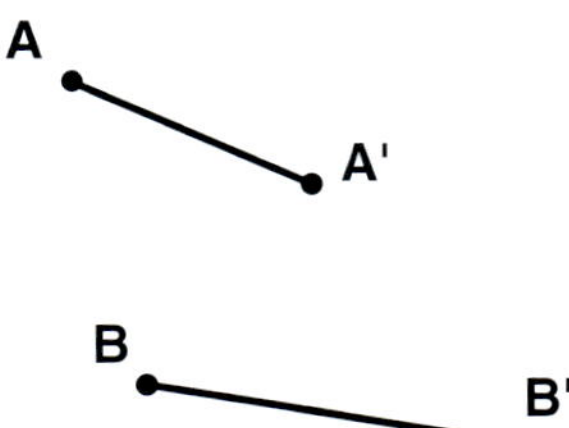

Fig. 3. Line segments A-A' and B-B' indicate the net movement of points A and B to A' and B'.

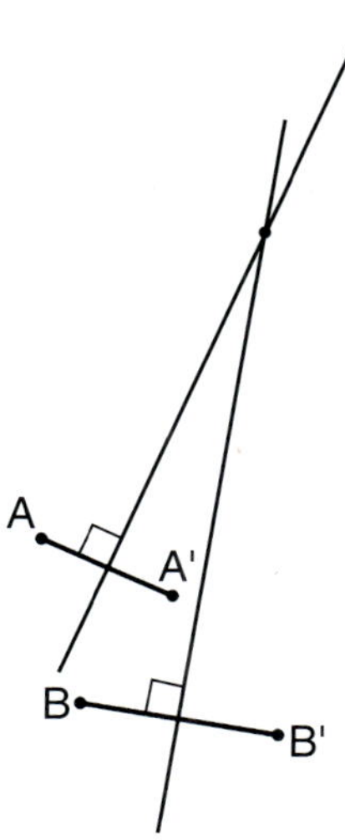

Fig. 4. **Perpendicular bisectors** of line segments A-A' and B-B' have been constructed. These perpendicular bisectors intersect each other at a point.

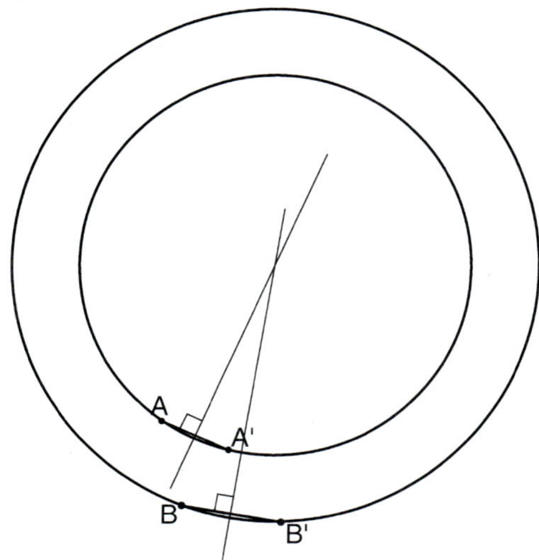

Fig. 5. The point of intersection of perpendicular bisectors of line segments A-A' and B-B' is the center of **concentric circles**, of which A-A' and B-B' are **chords**.

different lines can bisect a given line segment. They all lie in a ***perpendicularly bisecting plane*** (Fig. 7).

As is true for lines in two-dimensional space, in three-dimensional Euclidean space, any two planes are either parallel or intersect; there are no other alternatives. Flat planes intersect at a straight **line of intersection**. In Euclidean three-dimensional space, the exhaustive inventory of the ways in which two lines relate to each other is more complex than it is in two dimensions. Such lines can be ***parallel***, they can ***intersect***, or they can be ***nonparallel*** and ***nonintersecting*** (Fig. 8). Parallel lines and intersecting lines share the property of being coplanar (ie, they lie in the same plane). Lines that are neither parallel nor intersecting are always ***non-coplanar*** (ie, they cannot be drawn in the same two-dimensional plane).

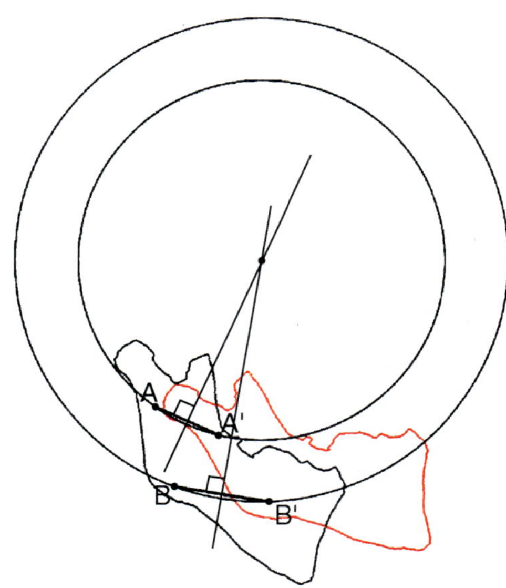

Fig. 6. The center point of the concentric circles is the **axis** about which the net movement of the mandibular tracings has occurred.

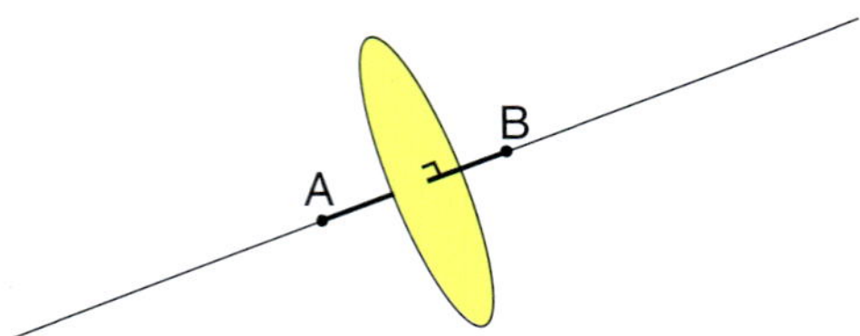

Fig. 7. Whereas a line segment in two-dimensional space has only one perpendicular bisector, a line segment in three-dimensional space has an infinity of perpendicular bisectors, all of which occupy a **perpendicularly bisecting plane**.

Considering the perpendicularly bisecting planes of line segments in three-dimensional space

Let us consider planes that bisect line segments at right angles in three-dimensional space. *In the case of parallel lines*, the perpendicularly bisecting planes are also parallel (Fig. 9). *In the case of line segments, the extensions of which intersect*, the perpendicularly bisecting planes also intersect to form a line of intersection. Because the line segments under discussion are coplanar, the two perpendicular bisectors of these segments that meet the line of intersection of the bisecting planes at ***right angles*** do so at the ***same point*** (Figs. 10 and 11). *In the case of line segments, the extensions of which are nonparallel and nonintersecting*, the perpendicularly bisecting planes of such segments also intersect to form a line of intersection. Because the line segments are non-coplanar, however, perpendicular bisectors of these segments that meet the line of intersection of the bisecting planes at right angles do so at ***two separate points*** (Fig. 12). *Unfortunately, it is impossible to represent adequately these circumstances in a two-dimensional diagram because of the non-coplanar nature of lines that are neither parallel nor intersecting. One would need special graphics and three-dimensional glasses.*

The three foregoing descriptions exhaust all possibilities

The reader should note that the *line of intersection of bisecting planes* is an ***axis of rotation*** (*the three-dimensional analog of a center of rotation in two-dimensional space*) about which the net movement of a solid object occurs.

Movements of solid objects in three-dimensional space

By applying the previously mentioned geometric considerations to a solid object that moves in three-dimensional space from an initial position to a final position, the net movement of the object can be represented by the coordinates of any landmarks, much as was the case in two dimensions. It takes three non-colinear points (A, B, and C) to fix a solid object (eg, a mandible) in three-dimensional space. Non-colinear points are ones that form a triangle and thus define a plane. (Colinear points would not do because the object would not be fully constrained and could rotate around such a line as an axis.) The coordinates of A, B, and C define an object in its

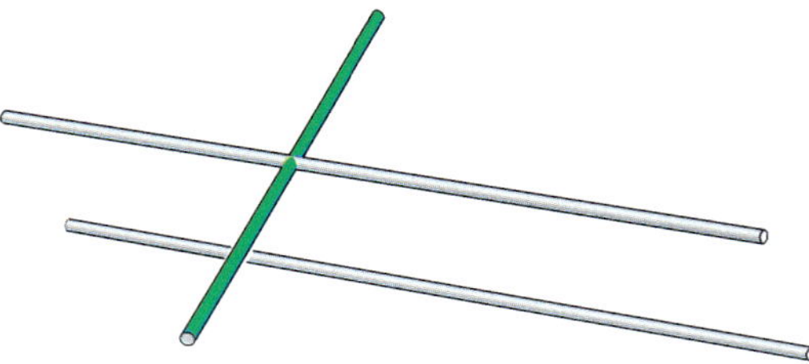

Fig. 8. This figure is meant to represent the three ways in which lines can relate to one another in three-dimensional space. They can be **parallel**, they can **intersect**, or they can be **nonparallel and nonintersecting**. There are no other alternatives. Note that parallel lines and intersecting lines are coplanar (ie, they can be represented in a single two-dimensional plane), whereas lines that are nonparallel and nonintersecting cannot be represented in a two-dimensional plane and are **non-coplanar**.

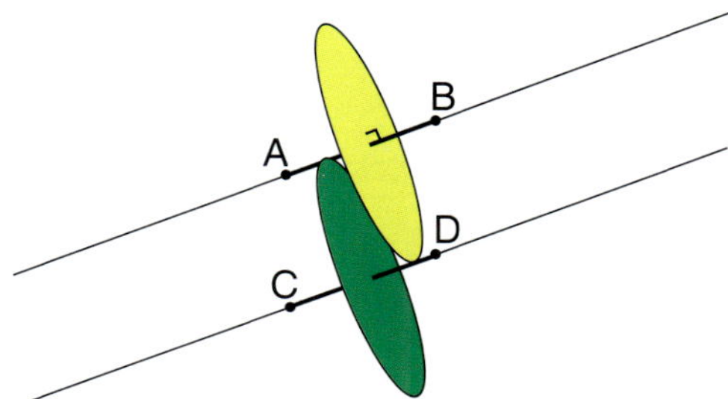

Fig. 9. Coplanar line segments that are parallel have parallel perpendicularly bisecting planes.

initial position, and those of A', B', and C' define the final position. The geometric relationship between any pair of the line segments A-A', B-B', and C-C' must conform to one of the descriptions in the previous discussion. Those descriptions comprehensively describe the net movement of solid objects in three-dimensional space. Line segments A-A', B-B', and C-C' are chords of ***concentric cylinders*** that share a common axis, analogous to the chords of circles in two-dimensional space, as discussed previously (Fig. 11).

Parameters of movement

The simplest comprehensive description of the net movement of a solid object in space states that it follows a ***helical path*** (similar to the thread of a screw) on the surface of a cylinder,

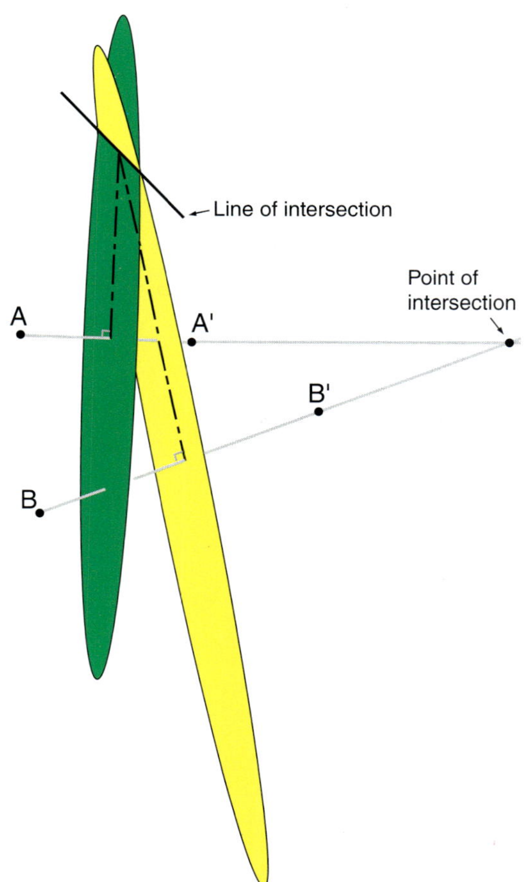

Fig. 10. Coplanar line segments, the extensions of which **intersect** at a point, have intersecting perpendicularly bisecting planes that interpenetrate each other at a **line of intersection**. In this instance, the perpendicular bisectors of line segments A-A' and B-B' that meet the line of intersection of planes at a right angles do so at a **common point**.

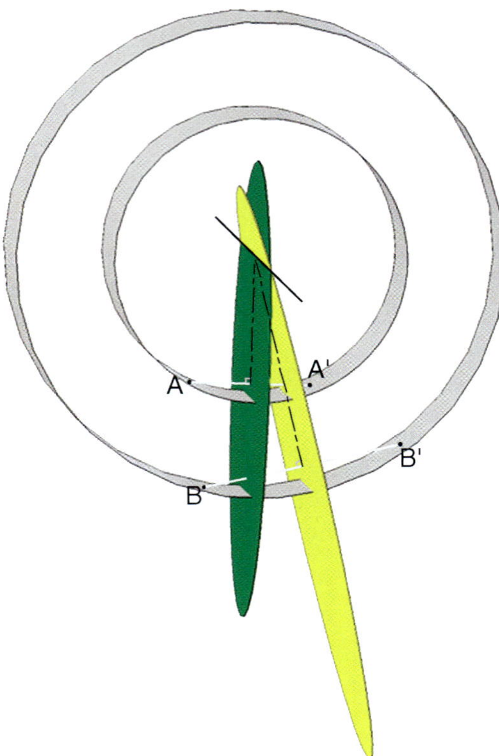

Fig. 11. The line of intersection of planes in Fig. 10 is the center line of **concentric cylinders**, of which line segments A-A' and B-B' are chords. If A-A' and B-B' are landmarks on a solid object moving in three-dimensional space, then such a center line is the axis or rotation about which the net movement between initial and final positions takes place.

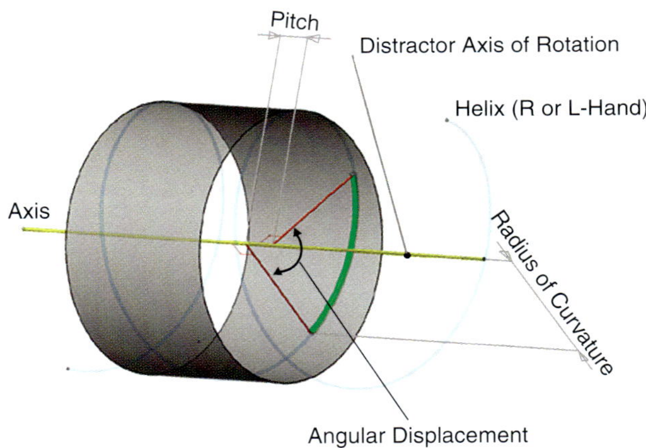

Fig. 12. Line segments that are nonparallel and nonintersecting also have perpendicularly bisecting planes that interpenetrate each other at a line of intersection. The perpendicular bisectors of these non-coplanar line segments that also meet the line of intersection of planes at right angles do so at different points because they also are non-coplanar. By definition, it is hard to create a figure in two dimensions that does justice to non-coplanarity. Such a figure would resemble Fig. 10 but with extensions of A-A' and B-B' that pass each other without intersecting and, as noted, perpendicular bisectors meting the line of intersection of planes at different points. For the sake of simplicity, this figure depicts the net movement of a single point on a solid object moving through three-dimensional space from an initial position to a final position.. The simplest depiction of such a path of movement is as a segment of a **helix** with a central axis of rotation. The **POM** includes the **location and orientation** of an axis in three-dimensional space, an **angular displacement**, and linear **translation** along the center line. (Angular displacement and linear translation determine the **pitch** of the helix, expressed alternatively as an angle or as the amount of translation accompanying a full rotation.) A helix also can be either **left** or **right handed**.

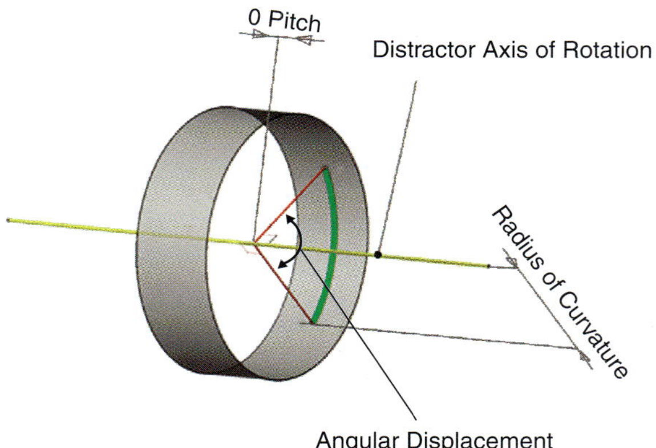

Fig. 13. Depiction of the POM for a simple rotation in a single plane (pitch equals zero). The other simple coplanar movement would be a simple translation parallel to a specified axis.

advancing as it rotates (Fig. 11). In describing any such movement, the following ***parameters of movement (POMs)*** are the essential descriptors (Figs. 12 and 13):

- The ***location and orientation*** of an axis of rotation
- The ***angular displacement*** about the axis
- The ***translation*** along the axis
- The ***handedness*** of the helical path (left or right)

In describing helices such as the threads of screws, parameters two and three are usually combined as ***pitch*** and frequently are expressed as the length of axial translation in one full circle of rotation around the axis or, alternatively, as a *pitch angle*.

Having identified an axis, if the translation of the object along the axis is zero, the movement is a ***pure rotation*** (Fig. 13). (This information corresponds to the second bulleted description.) If there is translation along the axis but angular displacement is zero, the movement is a ***pure translation***. (This information corresponds to the first bulleted description.) The most complex movements involve non-zero values for angular displacement and for translation and thus follow helical paths (Fig. 12). (This information corresponds to the third bulleted description.)

Pure translation and pure rotation are coplanar movements. That is, they can be described comprehensively in a single plane, whereas a helical path cannot. These facts are highly relevant to treatment planning modalities. Pure translational or pure rotational movements that occur in the sagittal plane of the head and neck are accurately portrayed in standard cephalometric X rays. This holds true when the bilateral symmetry of the face remains undisturbed, as it does in many of the surgically treated disturbances of mandibular and mid-facial growth, such as pure prognathism, retrognathism, and anterior open bite. Those disturbances of growth and development in which facial asymmetry is a dominant feature are not well represented in two-dimensional studies, such as Postero-Anterior (PA) and lateral cephalometric X rays, however. Such studies shed little useful light on the ***horizontal plane***, in which many important findings lie.

For clinical entities, such as condylar hyperplasia, hemifacial microsomia, and mandibular hemihypertrophy, neither the anatomy nor the required (helical) corrective movement can be represented adequately in a single planar image for reasons discussed previously. For such clinical entities, the gold standard has become the three-dimensional CT scan. The advent of the CT scan and the ability to use its database to perform three-dimensional reconstructions have led to a revolution in treatment-planning methodologies.

Treatment-planning considerations

Thinking about treatment planning in theoretical terms, if we digitize the positions of any three non-colinear points on a moving anatomic structure in initial and final positions, we can use a computerized treatment-planning system capable of manipulating three-dimensional data sets to calculate the POMs that define the desired corrective movement. It is a relatively straightforward next step to display such a movement in a segmented three-dimensional CT of the patient under study. With this capability, if we specify the position of a proposed osteotomy, the treatment planning system can (1) calculate and display the size and shape of an ostectomy specimen if there is an excess of bone and (2) calculate the size and shape of a bone graft, or a distraction gap, in cases in which there is deficient bone stock (Fig. 14).

When distraction osteogenesis is planned using the principles described previously, one can determine the POM for a proposed corrective movement. **The POM for such a correction, plus one additional variable controlled by the treatment planner, comprehensively defines the properties of a suitable distraction device that can—at least in theory—perform the desired movement following a fixed trajectory without mid-course corrections**. In addition to the POM, the surgeon or individual who conducts the treatment planning must identify the best anatomic location for distractor placement. The planned location of the distractor in relation to the axis of rotation determines of the **radius of curvature** of the requisite distraction device (Fig. 15).

The final implementation of a treatment plan (and the most fragile link in the chain) requires that the POM be exported to a **navigation** device in the operating room that enables the surgical team to place a fixed trajectory distraction device in the precise position that was determined in the treatment-planning process. This placement requires precise superimposition of the axis of curvature of the distractor on the calculated axis from the treatment plan, moving from the virtual world of the computer to the actual surgical field. The navigation device serves to relate the three-dimensional spatial coordinates of the axis of rotation to reliable anatomic landmarks within the surgical field.

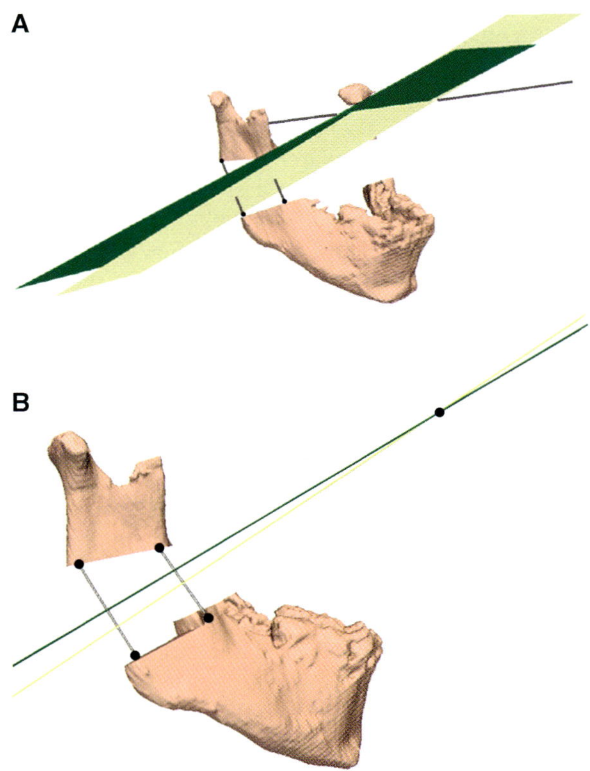

Fig. 14. (*A*) An oblique three-dimensional reconstruction of a mandible from a CT data set. The mandible has been segmented in a manner intended to simulate a proposed osteotomy cut intended to allow distraction osteogenesis. The condylar segment retains its original position, whereas the distal, tooth-bearing segment has been repositioned to occlude with the maxillary dentition (not shown). Yellow and green planes perpendicularly bisect the paths of motion of two reference points moving with the distal segment. The intersection of these two planes defines an axis of rotation about which the net corrective movement occurs. (*B*) The simulation has been reoriented to make the axis of rotation perpendicular to the plane of the page. The corrective movement is a simple rotation in a parasagittal plane.

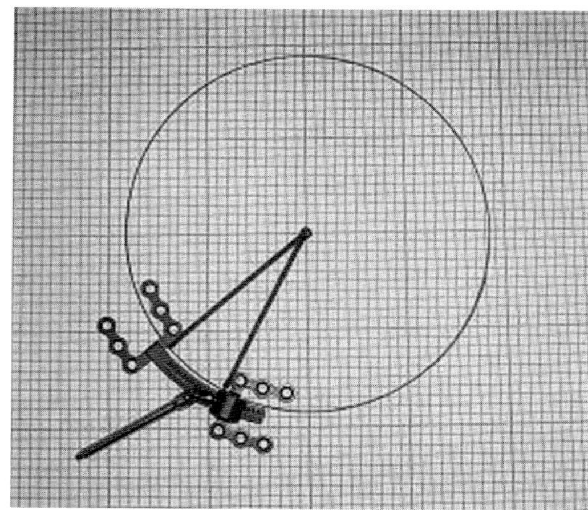

Fig. 15. A prototypical fixed trajectory, semi-buried distractor (Synthes Maxillofacial Paoli, Pennsylvania) superimposed on a diagram of POM for a simple rotational correction of a symmetrical deformity. The axis of the corrective movement is seen along with two radii of curvature delimiting the length of the distractive movement along a curvilinear path.

Navigation devices and methodologies currently are rapidly evolving. A comprehensive treatment of this highly specialized topic is beyond the scope of this article.

Persistent problems

Despite the wealth of anatomic information made available by CT scans and three-dimensional reconstructions, standard two-dimensional cephalometry remains the mainstay of orthodontic assessment. Cost and convenience are factors in the limited penetration of the orthodontic market by CT scanning.

It is technically difficult to integrate these two technologies. The data from one do not merge well with data from the other. They are like different languages without a convenient "Rosetta stone" to aid in translation. There is an enormous body of information on growth and development and on normative cephalometric indices in the orthodontic literature that one would like to use while treatment planning in the three-dimensional CT realm. Unfortunately, it remains difficult to identify standard cephalometric landmarks on CT scans. Many landmarks on a cephalogram are artifacts of superimposition and do not correspond to anatomy as depicted in a CT scan. It is possible, however, that refinements in the technique of "***volume rendering***" may make it possible to simulate a cephalogram from CT data to develop cephalometric standards and display such landmarks on a three-dimensional reconstruction.

Integration of information regarding occlusion

Occlusal considerations are not well elucidated by CT scans thus far. The occlusion itself or dental models remain the best source of the occlusal data requisite to precise treatment planning. It is desirable to obtain occlusal data in a digital format from the teeth themselves or from dental models of the teeth and to import these data into the treatment planning system. We have attempted this on a trial basis using articulated dental models and locking templates that capture initial and final occlusal positions and using a mechanical digitizer (Fig. 16).

Currently, it is possible to obtain a digital occlusal data set by means of laser scanning articulated dental models or the teeth themselves. This is a promising potential addition to the overall treatment-planning armamentarium.

Integration of soft-tissue facial surface anatomy

One of the most useful additions to treatment planning would be the ability to integrate—in a digital format—data regarding soft-tissue facial anatomy obtained from photographic images

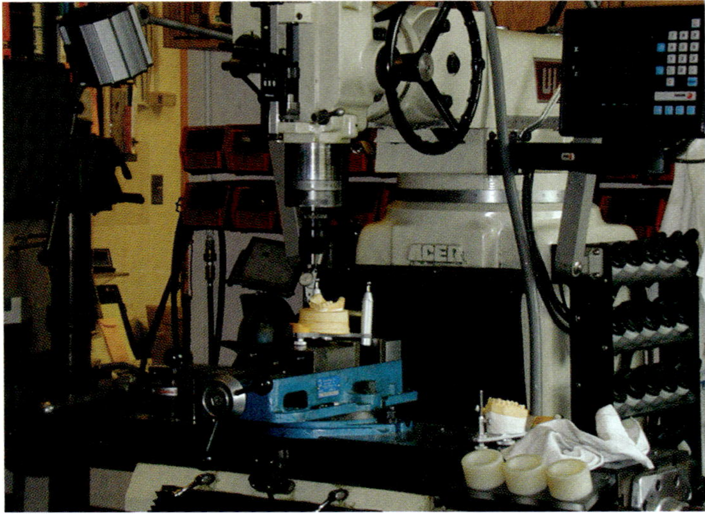

Fig. 16. Experimental measurement of the dental landmarks in three-dimensional space using a milling machine digital readout. The spatial coordinates of the initial and final positions of three landmarks on the models capture accurate occlusal data, which can be used to guide segmentation of a three-dimensional CT of the patient by a treatment-planning program.

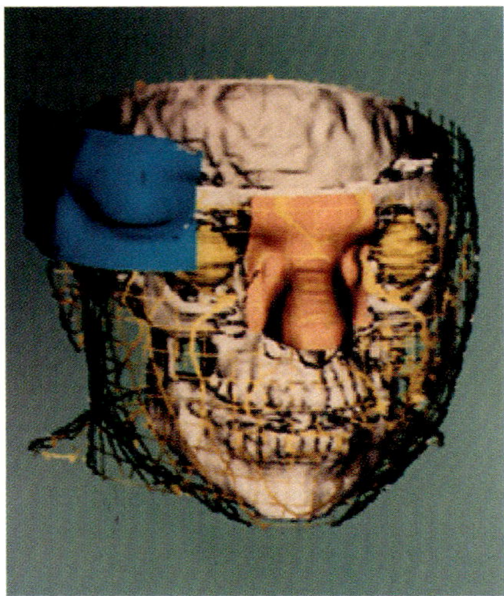

Fig. 17. An early, seminal effort to display soft-tissue and skeletal anatomy on the same three-dimensional CT reconstruction. (Courtesy of David Altobelli, DMD, MD, Hollis, NH.)

or from CT data sets (Fig. 17). With a library of data on pre- and postoperative skeletal anatomy and soft-tissue surface anatomy with which to work, eventually it should be possible to simulate accurately the esthetic consequence of proposed skeletal movements.

Summary

To provide an optimal service for patients, the surgeon of the future will require greater fluency in mathematics, computer science, and other areas of technology. The pace of this trend is likely to accelerate.

Further readings

Altobelli DE. Computer-assisted three-dimensional planning for cranio-maxillofacial surgery: selected readings in oral and maxillofacial surgery. Dallas: University of Texas SW Medical Center; 1994. p. 1–36.

Altobelli DE, Kikinis R, Mulliken JB, et al. Computer-assisted three-dimensional planning in craniofacial surgery. Plast Reconstr Surg 1993;92:576–85.

Coxeter HSM. Regular polytopes. New York: Dover Publications, Inc.; 1973.

Everett PC, Seldin EB, Troulis MJ, et al., A 3-D system for planning and simulating minimally-invasive distraction osteogenesis of the facial skeleton. In: Delp SI, Digioia AM, Jaramaz B, editors. Proceedings of the 3rd International Conference on Medical Image Computing and Computer-Assisted Intervention (MICCAI). New York: Springer-Verlag; 2000. p. 1029–33.

Gleick. J. Chaos. New York: Penguin Books, Inc.; 1987.

Lang S, Murrow G. Geometry. 2nd edition. New York: Springer-Verlag; 1988.

Livio M. The golden ratio. New York: Broadway Books; 2002.

Schneider MS. A beginner's guide to constructing the universe. New York: HarperCollins Publishers; 1994.

Seldin EB, Troulis MJ, Kaban LB. Evaluation of a semi-buried, fixed-trajectory, curvilinear distraction device in an animal model. J Oral Maxillofac Surg 1999;57(12):1442–6.

Trauner R. Kiefer- und gesichtschirurgie. Munich: Urban and Schwarzenberg; 1973.

Williams R. The geometrical foundation of natural structure. New York: Dover Publications, Inc.; 1979.

ELSEVIER
SAUNDERS

Atlas Oral Maxillofacial Surg Clin N Am 13 (2005) 25–39

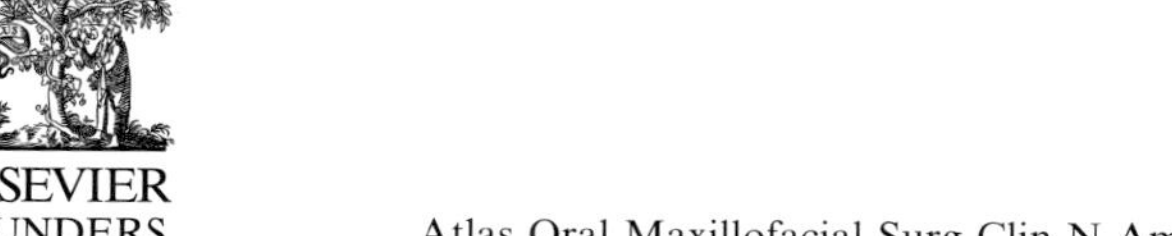

Atlas of the Oral and Maxillofacial Surgery Clinics

Three-Dimensional Computer-Aided Surgical Simulation for Maxillofacial Surgery

James J. Xia, MD, PhD[a,b,*], Jaime Gateno, DDS, MD[a], John F. Teichgraeber, MD, FACS[b]

[a]*Department of Oral and Maxillofacial Surgery, Dental Branch, The University of Texas Health Science Center, 6516 MD Anderson Boulevard, Suite DBB 2.059, Houston, TX 77030, USA*

[b]*Division of Pediatric Surgery, Department of Surgery, Medical School, The University of Texas Health Science Center, Houston, TX 77030, USA*

Problems of current surgical planning methods for craniomaxillofacial surgery

The current methods used to plan craniomaxillofacial surgery vary according to the type of surgery that is being planned. Generally, the planning process involves the following steps. The first step is to gather data from different sources. These sources include physical examination, medical photographs, and medical imaging studies that include plain radiographs, cephalometric radiographs, CT, and other studies. When the surgery involves the jaws, it is also necessary to use plaster dental models, which are mounted on a dental articulator. The surgeons will then use these data to create a complete picture of the condition. This task is often difficult, especially in patients with complex three-dimensional (3D) problems.

The second step in the planning process is to simulate the surgery. In craniomaxillofacial surgery, this step may begin with prediction tracings. The surgical simulation is completed by moving the bone tracings to the desired position. A drawback of prediction tracing is that it is two-dimensional. As a result, with this technique, it is impossible to simulate surgery in three-dimensions. Although, 3D CT images have been useful in allowing the surgeons to visualize the patient's condition, the images have not been particularly useful for surgical simulation. The software packages currently available do not have the necessary tools to allow for surgical simulation. Another problem with plain radiographs or CTs is that they do not render the teeth with the accuracy that is necessary for surgical simulation. For these reasons, surgeries that involve the jaws are also simulated on plaster dental models that have been mounted on an articulator. This is accomplished by cutting the dental models into pieces and repositioning them in the desired location. The purpose of this step is to establish a new dental occlusion and to fabricate surgical splints. A drawback of plaster dental models is that they do not depict the surrounding bony structures. Therefore, it is impossible for the surgeon to visualize the skeletal changes that occur during model surgery, which is critical in the treatment of complex craniomaxillofacial deformities.

Another means of simulating surgery is the use of CT-based physical models produced by rapid prototyping techniques (eg, stereolithography [STL]). Although these models are useful, they have several disadvantages. One disadvantage is that the teeth are not accurate enough for

This work was partially supported by NIH grant 1 R41 DE 016171-01, UCRC (UT–Houston Medical School) grant M01RR002558, and Stryker-Leibinger.

* Corresponding author. Department of Oral and Maxillofacial Surgery, Dental Branch, The University of Texas Health Science Center at Houston, 6516 MD Anderson Boulevard, Suite DBB 2.059, Houston, TX 77030.

E-mail address: James.J.Xia@uth.tmc.edu (J.J. Xia).

1061-3315/05/$ - see front matter
doi:10.1016/j.cxom.2004.10.004

precise surgical simulation of cases involving the occlusion. This is because the CT image data from which models are built are subject to artifacts resulting from metallic implants often present in the patient's teeth. Another disadvantage is that it is impossible to simulate different surgeries on a single model. Once the model is cut, it is impossible to undo the cut. Another disadvantage is that these models can be fairly expensive.

The final step in the surgical planning process is the transfer of the surgical plan to the operating room. In cases involving the jaws, this is done by using dental splints. These splints help the surgeon place the jaws in the desired position. In cases that do not involve the dentition, surgeons currently do not have an accurate method of transferring the plan to the operating room. Certain measurements taken during the planning process can be used to guide surgery, but the placement of the bones in the desire position is more of an art than a science.

As surgeons, our goal is to create a surgical plan that will result in an ideal surgical outcome. The problems discussed above greatly limit the accuracy of the surgical plan. Therefore, the Surgical Planning Laboratory at the University of Texas Houston Health Science Center has developed various applications for 3D computer-aided surgical simulation (CASS).

Computer-aided surgical simulation in complex orthognathic surgery

The current planning methods used in orthognathic surgery are clinically acceptable because most patients require relatively simple operations. However, it is well known that these methods are less than accurate. In these patients, minor inaccuracies in the surgical plan are not critical because the clinical outcomes are usually acceptable. Current surgical planning methods are not adequate for the treatment of patients with complex maxillofacial deformities (eg, hemifacial microsomia). In these types of patients, it is not uncommon to have unwanted outcomes. It is the authors' opinion that in patients with complex maxillofacial deformities CASS significantly improves the accuracy of the surgical plan and enhances the surgeon's ability to accurately reproduce the plan at the time of surgery.

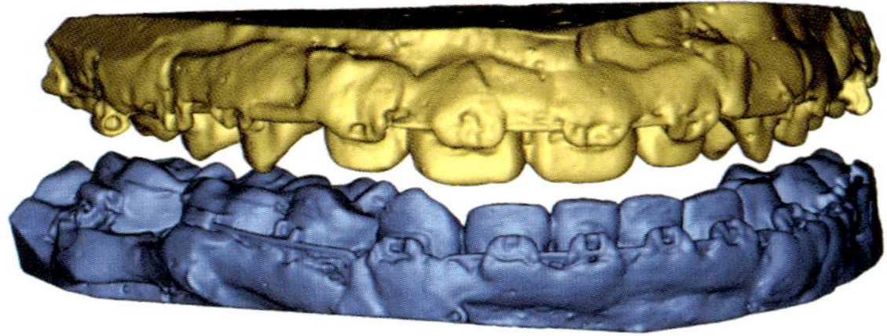

Fig. 1. Maxillary and mandibular digital dental models. (See text relating to this figure on page 5.)

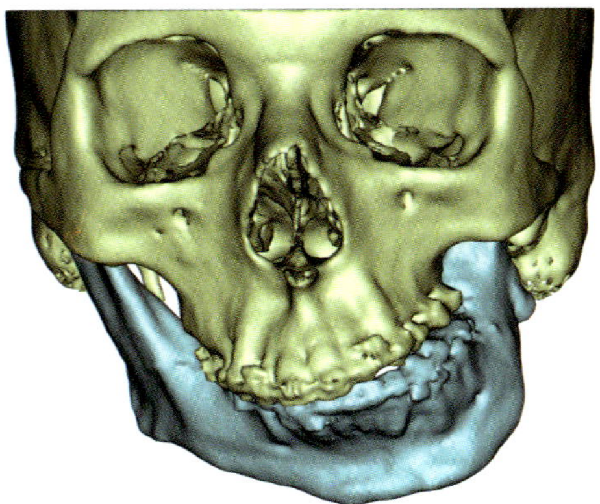

Fig. 2. The CT images are segmented and reconstructed to create separate models of the midface and the mandible. (See text relating to this figure on page 5.)

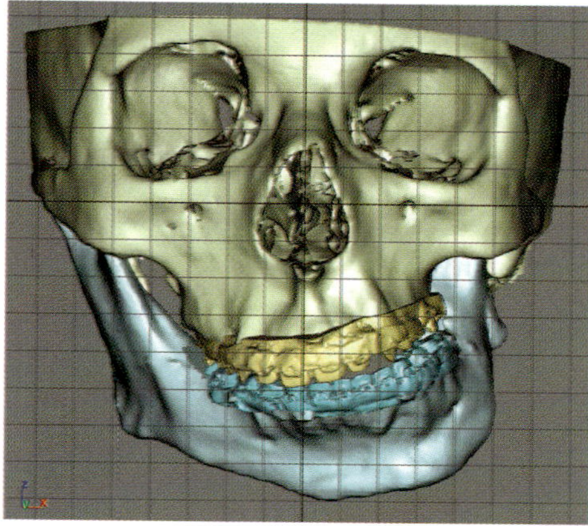

Fig. 3. A computerized composite skull model, which is oriented to the natural head position, reproduces both the bony structures and the dentition with a high degree of accuracy. (See text relating to this figure on page 5.)

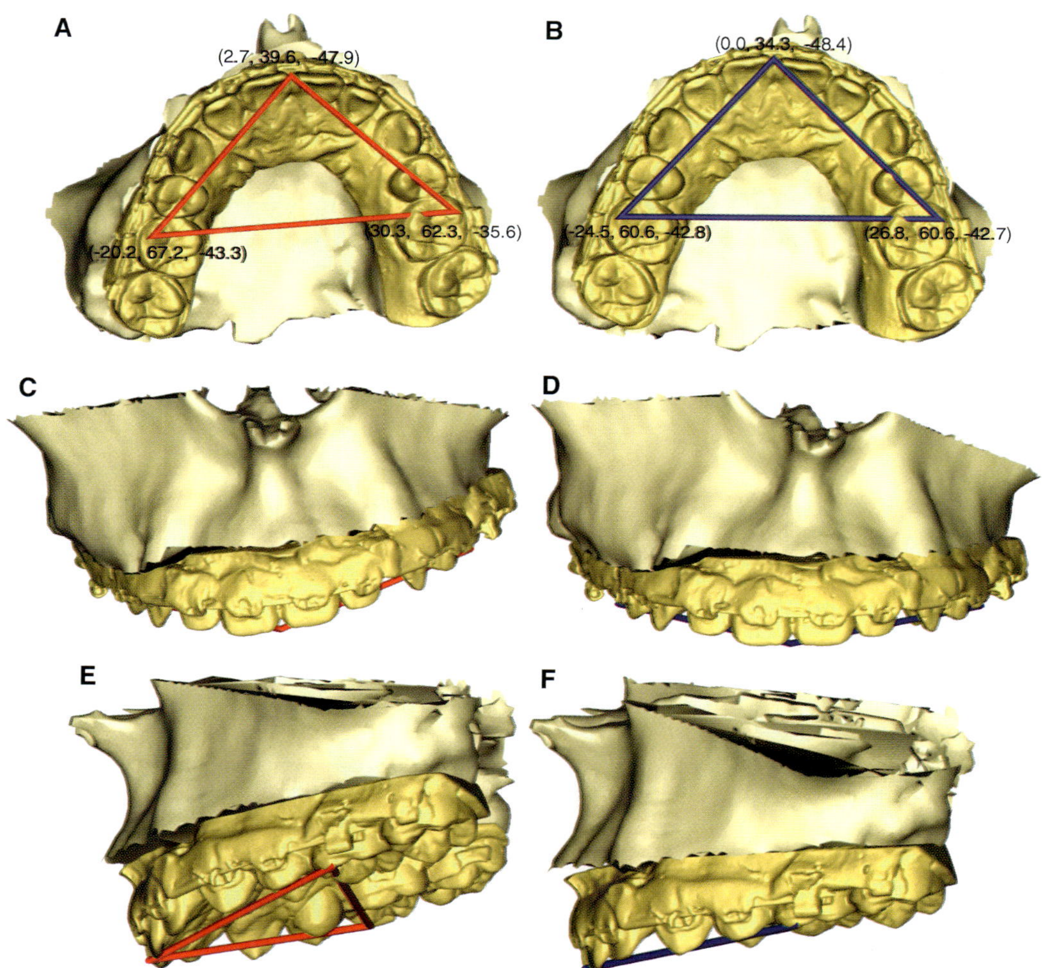

Fig. 4. Three points are digitized on the maxillary dentition, forming a red triangle. One of the points is placed on the maxillary midline and other two on the mesiobuccal cusps of the maxillary right and left first molars. The computer automatically records the x, y, and z coordinates for these points. Using these coordinates, the planning system will move the triangle to the desired position to correct the pitch, yaw, and roll of the maxilla. The triangle at the desired position is colored blue. (*A*, *C*, *E*) The bottom, frontal, and left views of the maxilla are shown at the original position. (*B*, *D*, *F*) The bottom, frontal, and left views are shown of the maxilla after its pitch, yaw, and roll are corrected. (See text relating to this figure on page 6.)

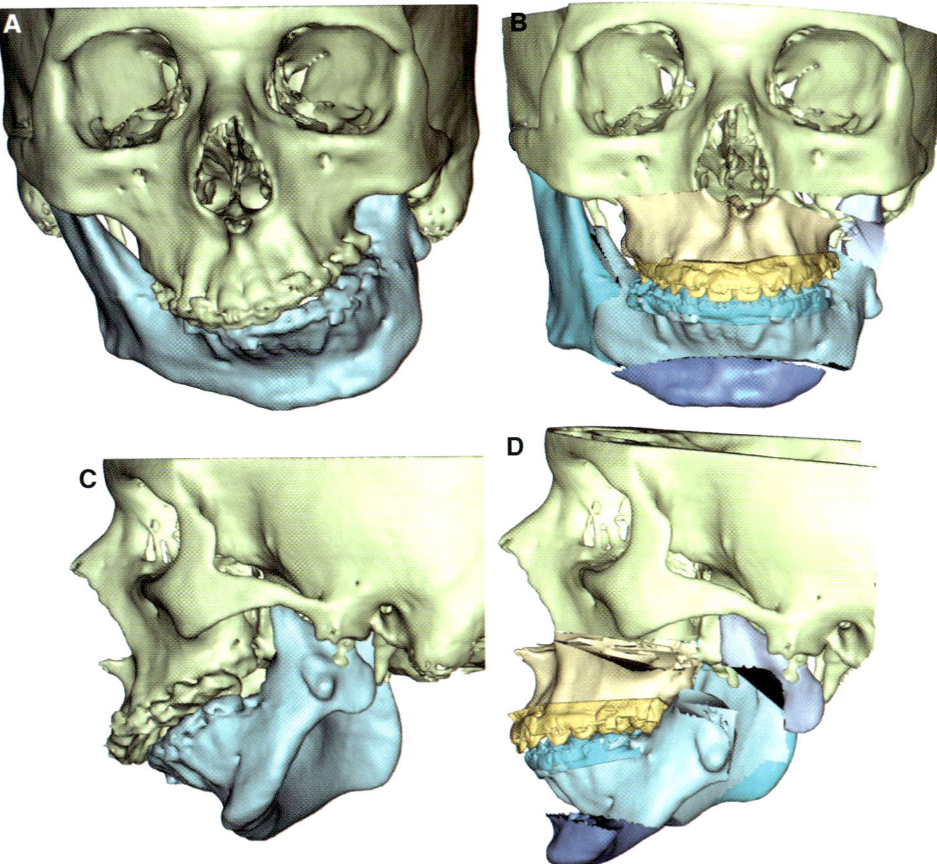

Fig. 5. (*A*, *C*) Frontal and left views of a patient's model are shown before computer simulation. (*B*, *D*) Frontal and left views of the same patient's model are shown after simulation. The simulated surgery includes a Le Fort I osteotomy, a right sagittal split ramus osteotomy, a left inverted L ramus osteotomy, and a genioplasty. (See text relating to this figure on page 6.)

Creation of a computerized composite skull model

Current CASS systems use CT images as the source of data. Computed tomography is excellent for representing bones. However, it is not capable of accurately reproducing the teeth to the degree that is necessary for surgical planning. This is because CT scanners capture images layer by layer. Data between the image layers are missing and are reconstructed by mathematical algorithms. Currently, the most precise CT scanners scan at a minimum interval

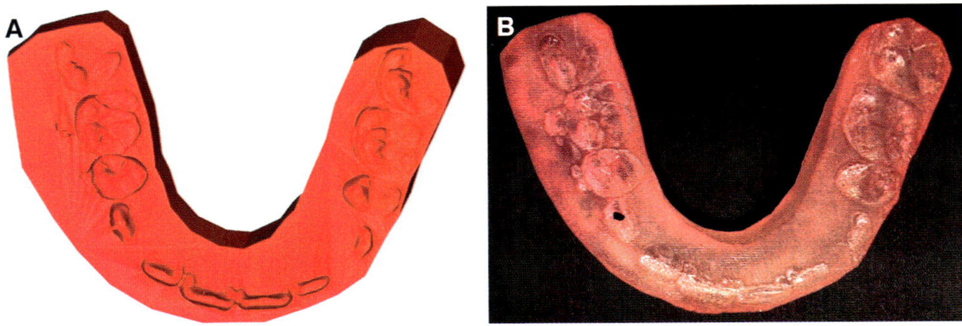

Fig. 6. (*A*) The digital surgical splint that is created in the computer is shown in comparison with the physical surgical splint that is created by a rapid prototyping machine (Medical Modeling LLC, Golden, Colorado) (*B*). (See text relating to this figure on page 6.)

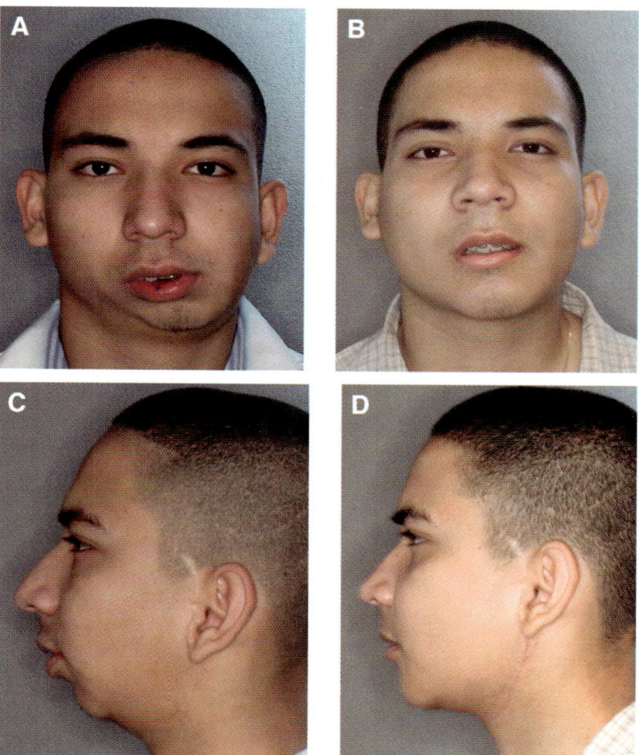

Fig. 7. A comparison of the patient before and after the surgery. (*A, C*) Preoperative photographs of a patient. (*B, D*) Postoperative photographs of the patient in whom the authors' technique was used. (See text relating to this figure on page 6.)

of 0.625 mm. This scanning interval does not reproduce the teeth accurately. Furthermore, it is difficult if not impossible to remove scattering, which is caused by metal orthodontic brackets or dental restorations. Because of these limitations, current 3D CT-based surgical planning systems for orthognathic surgery still relay on conventional plaster dental model surgery to establish the occlusion and to fabricate the surgical splints.

Plaster dental models mounted on articulators are the most accurate replicas of the patient's teeth. Nonetheless, these models lack bony support. The limitation of conventional dental model surgery is that the planner cannot visualize the surrounding bony structures, which are critical in the treatment of complex craniofacial deformities. To this end, the authors have developed a technique for creating a computerized composite skull model and have demonstrated its accuracy.

The "composite skull model" consists of a set of digital dental models that has been incorporated into a 3D CT model of the craniofacial structures. Regular plaster dental models are scanned in a highly accurate 3D scanner (accuracy of 0.1 mm), creating maxillary and mandibular digital dental models (Fig. 1) (Figure 1 located on page 2 of this article.). A regular CT scan of the patient's craniofacial skeleton is obtained with a slice thickness of 1.2 mm. The CT images are segmented and reconstructed, creating separate models of the midface and the mandible (Fig. 2) (Figure 2 located on page 2 of this article.). The digital dental models are merged with the 3D CT models, resulting in a computerized composite skull model (Fig. 3) (Figure 3 located on page 3 of this article.). This computerized model reproduces both the bony structures and the dentition with a high degree of accuracy.

Quantification of the deformity and surgical simulation

After the computerized composite skull model has been generated, it is necessary to orient the model to the natural head position (see Fig. 3) and to complete a cephalometric analysis.

The purpose of the cephalometric analysis step is to quantify the deformity. Once this quantification has been completed, the surgeon can proceed with surgical simulation. Using this system, the surgeon is able to simulate an operation as if it was being performed in the operating room. The operator can perform virtual osteotomies and move the bony segments to the desired position.

In patients requiring bimaxillary surgery, the maxillary osteotomy is usually completed first. The task of repositioning the maxilla to the desired position may require complex movements and rotations (transformations). During conventional surgical planning, most surgeons use Erickson's model table to complete this task. This process can be laborious and time consuming. To solve this problem, our laboratory has developed a technique to reposition the maxilla in 3D space. In this technique, three points are digitized on the maxillary dentition, forming a triangle. One of the points is placed on the maxillary midline, and other two points are placed on the mesiobuccal cusps of the maxillary right and left first molars (Fig. 4a) (Figure 4 located on page 3 of this article.). The computer will then automatically record the x, y, and z coordinates for these points. Using these coordinates, the planning system will correct the pitch, yaw, and roll of the maxilla (see Fig. 4). Afterward, the surgeon moves the maxilla in the anteroposterior and vertical directions as required. Fig. 5 (Figure 5 located on page 4 of this article.) shows a patient's model before and after computer simulation. The simulated surgery includes a Le Fort I osteotomy, a right sagittal split ramus osteotomy, a left inverted L ramus osteotomy, and a genioplasty.

Transfer of the computerized surgical plan in the operating room

Once the ideal treatment plan has been established, the surgeon needs to reproduce it at the time of surgery. It is the authors' opinion that for a CASS system to be useful, it should have the necessary tools to allow the transfer of the plan at the time of surgery. Time spent developing a computerized treatment plan would be worthless if the plan cannot be reproduced on the patient. For this reason, our laboratory has developed methods to fabricate surgical splints using computer-aided designing/computer-aided manufacturing techniques (Fig. 6) (Figure 6 located on page 4 of this article.). These methods eliminate the need to fabricated splints by hand on plaster dental models. Fig. 7 (Figure 7 located on page 5 of this article.) shows pre- and postoperative photographs of a patient in whom this technique was used.

Computer-aided surgical simulation in temporomandibular joint reconstruction

Treatment of bony ankylosis of the temporomandibular joint (TMJ) poses a significant challenge to the surgeon. Complex and distorted anatomy with loss of anatomical landmarks

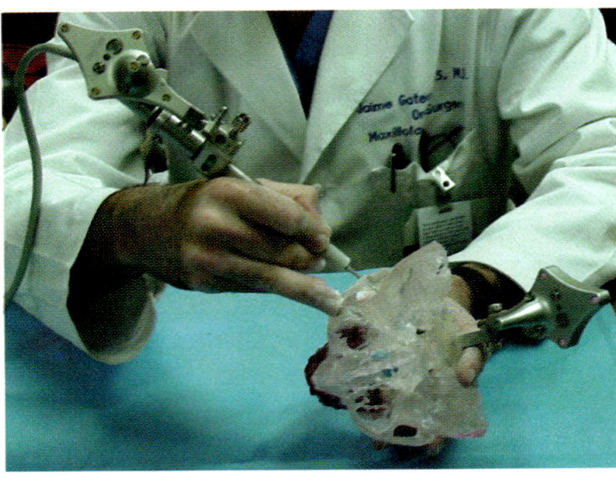

Fig. 8. The resection of the ankylosis and the preparation of the recipient site are simulated on an STL model before surgery, using a navigated drill. (See text relating to this figure on page 9.)

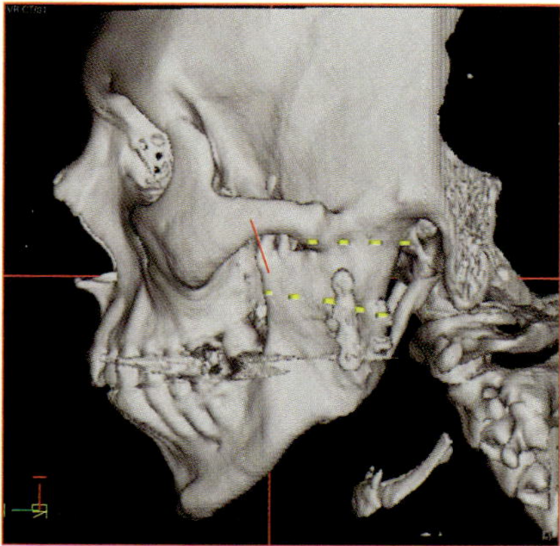

Fig. 9. The contour and location of the recipient sites on the simulated STL model are recorded in the navigation system. (See text relating to this figure on page 9.)

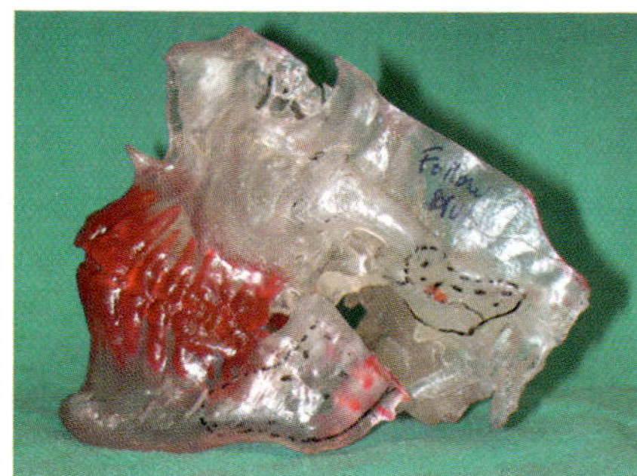

Fig. 10. A completed surgical simulation on the STL model. (See text relating to this figure on page 9.)

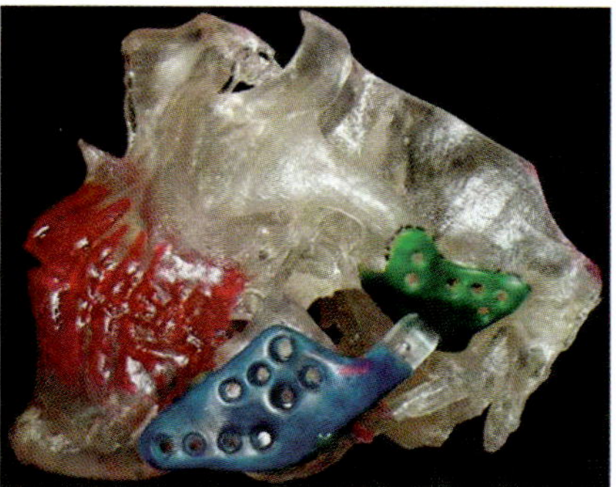

Fig. 11. A set of custom-made wax TMJ prosthesis models. (*Courtesy of* TMJ Implants, Inc., Golden, Colorado) (See text relating to this figure on page 9.)

makes TMJ reconstructive surgery particularly difficult. There are two steps in the treatment of TMJ bony ankylosis. The first step is to resect the ankylosis, thereby creating a critical size gap. The second step is to reconstruct the joint. Reconstruction can be completed using autogenous grafts or a prosthetic joint. Because of the altered anatomy, reconstruction using a custom-made prosthesis often requires two operations. In the first operation, the ankylosis is resected, and in the second operation the custom prosthesis is installed. After the first operation, an STL model is obtained from which the custom-made joint prosthesis is fabricated.

Using the CASS planning system and intraoperative navigation, the authors' team has been able to treat complex cases of TMJ bony ankylosis using custom-made prostheses in a single operation. Using this approach, the surgeon obtains an STL model before surgery. On this

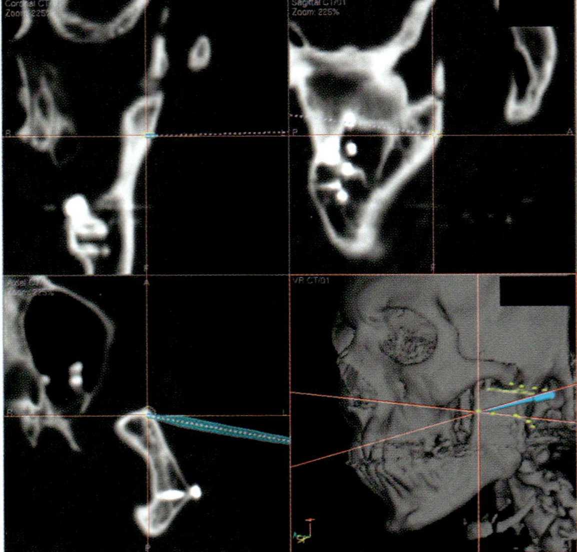

Fig. 12. At the time of surgery, the surgeon uses the navigation system to duplicate the planned resection and preparation of the recipient site on the patient. (See text relating to this figure on page 9.)

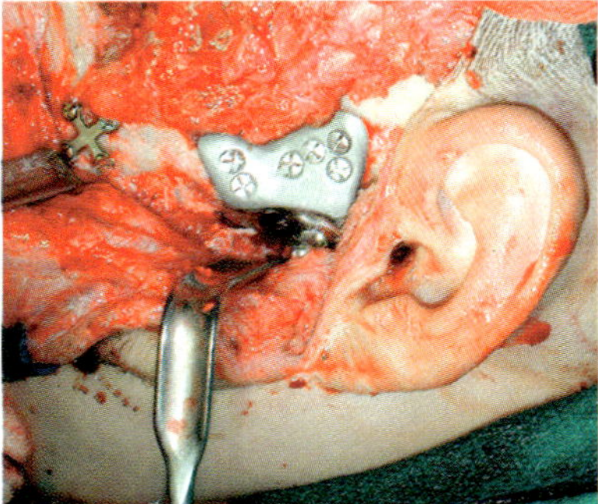

Fig. 13. The same TMJ prosthesis is installed on the recipient site. (See text relating to this figure on page 9.)

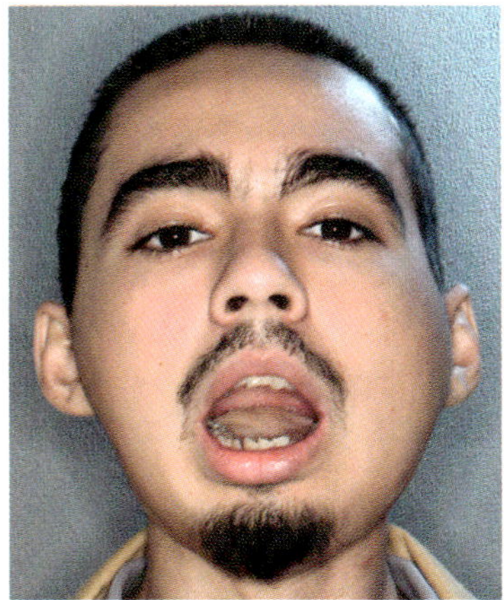

Fig. 14. Postoperative photograph 1 year after the surgery. (See text relating to this figure on page 9.)

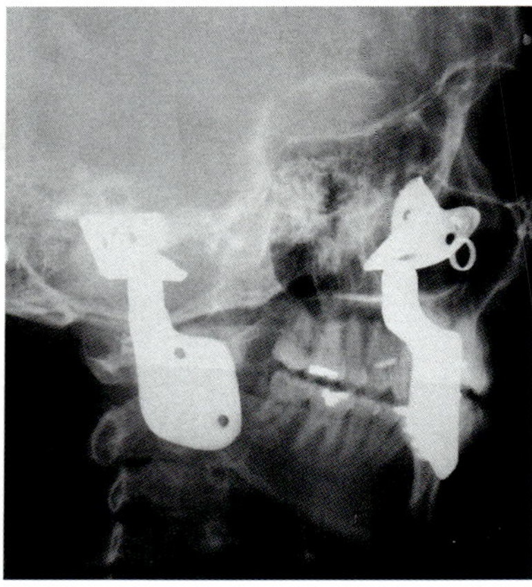

Fig. 15. Radiographs 1 year after the surgery. (See text relating to this figure on page 9.)

model, the resection of the ankylosis and the preparation of the recipient site are simulated using a navigated drill (Fig. 8) (Figure 8 located on page 6 of this article.). In addition, the contour and location of the recipient sites are recorded in the navigation system (Fig. 9) (Figure 9 located on page 7 of this article.). Once this is completed (Fig. 10) (Figure 10 located on page 7 of this article.), the custom-made prosthesis is fabricated on the STL model (TMJ Implants, Inc., Golden, Colorado) (Fig. 11) (Figure 11 located on page 7 of this article.). At the time of surgery, the surgeon uses the navigation system to duplicate the planned resection and preparation of the recipient site on the patient (Fig. 12) (Figure 12 located on page 8 of this article.). Moreover, the navigation system also helps the surgeon avoid important structures, for example, the internal maxillary artery. It has been the authors' experience that the use of this system greatly enhances the ability to treat these complex cases in a single operation (Figs. 13–15). (Figure 13–15 located on pages 8, 9 of this article.)

Computer-aided surgical simulation in distraction osteogenesis

Mandibular distraction

Distraction osteogenesis has been used to treat patients with different types of mandibular deformities. Currently, the most commonly accepted indication for mandibular distraction is the treatment of infants and children with severe mandibular hypoplasia. However, it is risky to go

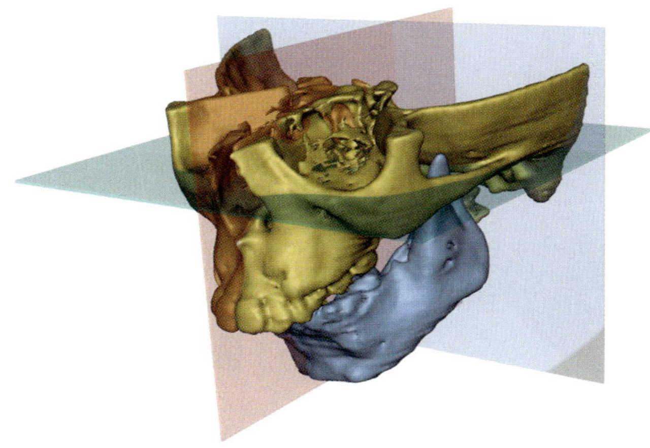

Fig. 16. The patient's computer models, including a facial skeletal and a mandibular model, are oriented in a unique 3D coordinate system. (See text relating to this figure on page 10.)

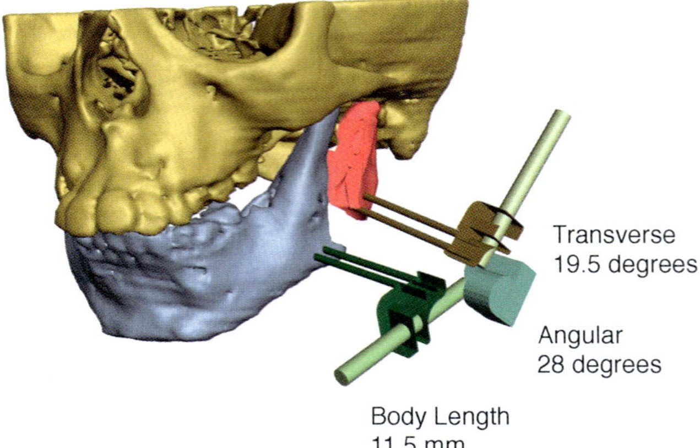

Fig. 17. Once a particular distractor is chosen, a virtual model of the distractor is created and installed. The process of distraction can then be simulated, and the computer software formulates the linear and angular changes for each of the distractor components needed to achieve the desired outcome. This establishes the recipe necessary to activate the device during the distraction process. (See text relating to this figure on page 11.)

to the operating room without a plan for the treatment of these patients. Traditional surgical planning methods, including the use of cephalometric tracing, acetate drawings, and plaster dental model surgery, are inadequate to solve the complex 3D problems involved in mandibular distraction. The best way to solve these complex problems is to use 3D CASS.

A CT scan of the patient's maxillofacial region is used. After the mandible is segmented from the remaining part of the skeleton on the axial CT slices, two 3D computer models, a facial skeletal model and a mandibular model, are created (Fig. 16) (Figure 16 located on page 9 of this article.). The models are then oriented in a unique 3D coordinate system (see Fig. 16). The osteotomies are performed, separating the mandible into proximal and distal segments. In bilateral cases, two osteotomies are performed, separating the mandible into one distal and two proximal segments.

An animation is created to simulate the movement of the distal segment. The purpose of this animation is to help the surgeon select the appropriate type of distractor. The selection of a particular type of device should be based on the ability of that device to perform the necessary spatial movements. The animation is similar to traditional animation used in cartoons, in which a series of still images (frames) are displayed sequentially to produce the illusion of motion. Using the animation software, it is only necessary to create the initial and final frames; all the necessary intermediate frames are created automatically. The first frame is the frame that shows the mandible in its preoperative condition. To create the last frame, the proximal and distal

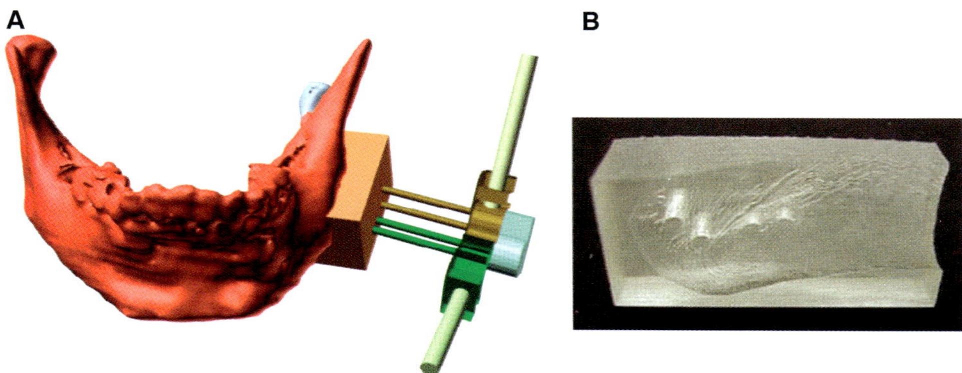

Fig. 18. The transfer of a simulated surgical plan is accomplished by creating a surgical template. (*A*) A digital template that is designed in the computer. (*B*) A physical template that is fabricated by a stereolithographic apparatus (Medical Modeling LLC, Golden, Colorado) (see Fig. 18b). (See text relating to this figure on page 12.)

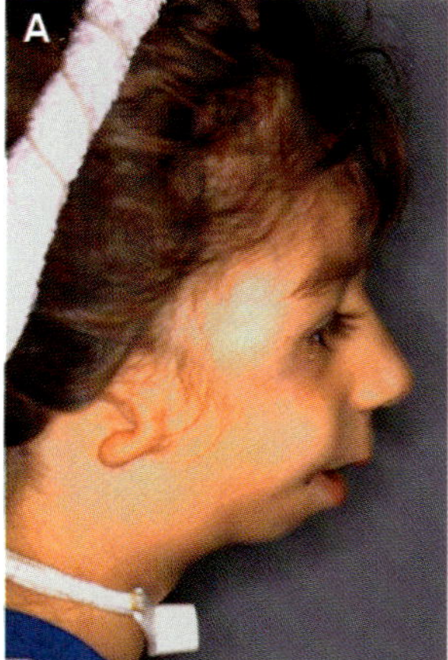

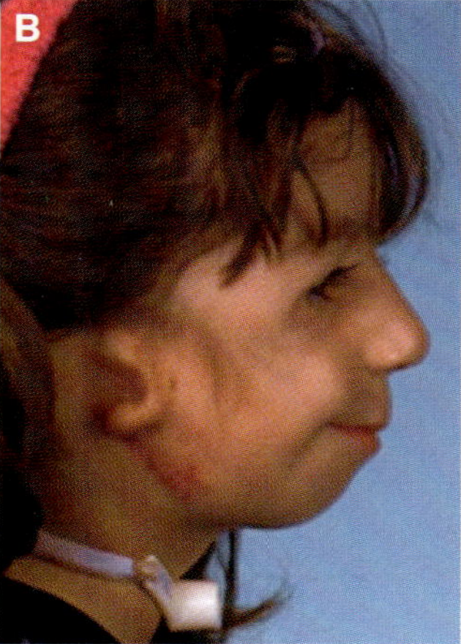

Fig. 19. A comparison of a patient before (*A*) and after (*B*) mandibular distraction. (See text relating to this figure on page 12.) (*From*: Gateno J, Teichgraeber FJ, Aguilar E. Computer planning for distraction osteogenesis. Plast Reconstr Surg 2000; 105(3):873–82.)

segments are mobilized to the desired final position. After the animation sequence has been created, it can be visualized from multiple angles.

Once the decision to use a particular distractor is made, a virtual model of the distractor is created and installed (Fig. 17) (Figure 17 located on page 10 of this article.). After the distractor is installed, the process of distraction can be simulated. In bilateral cases (eg, Treacher-Collins syndrome), the distal segment is moved to maximal intercuspation, while the condyles of the proximal segments remain in the glenoid fossae. In unilateral cases (eg, hemifacial microsomia), the distal segment is rotated around the uninvolved condyle until the chin and mandibular dental midlines are aligned with the sagittal plane. It is important to note that the movement of the distal segment is constrained by the distractor. Finally, the computer software formulates the linear and angular changes for each of the distractor components needed to achieve the desired outcome. This establishes the recipe necessary to activate the device during the distraction process (see Fig. 17).

The success of a planning process depends on the surgeon's ability to execute the plan at the time of surgery. As a result, the authors developed a technique that enables the precise installation of the distractor, as indicated in the presurgical plan. To accomplish this, it is necessary to transfer information regarding the position and orientation of the device from the

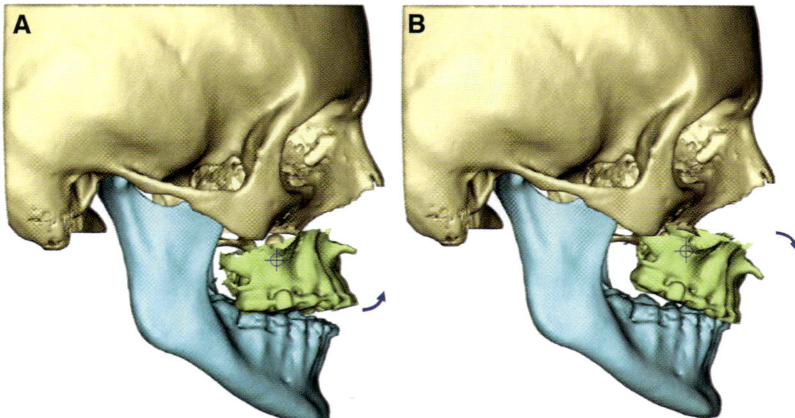

Fig. 20. The center of resistance (⊕) is defined as a point at which an applied force produces linear displacement without rotation. (*A*) If the force is applied below the center of resistance, a counterclockwise (*curved arrow*) rotation will be introduced, resulting in an anterior open bite. (*B*) If the force is applied above the center of resistance, a clockwise (*curved arrow*) rotation of the maxilla will be introduced, and the complication of anterior open bite can be prevented. (See text relating to this figure on page 13.)

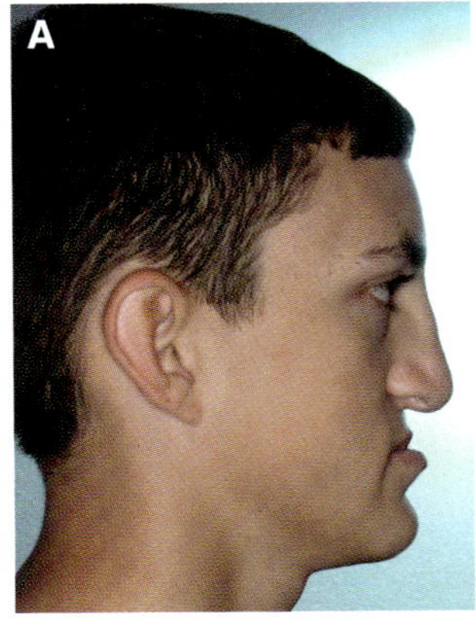

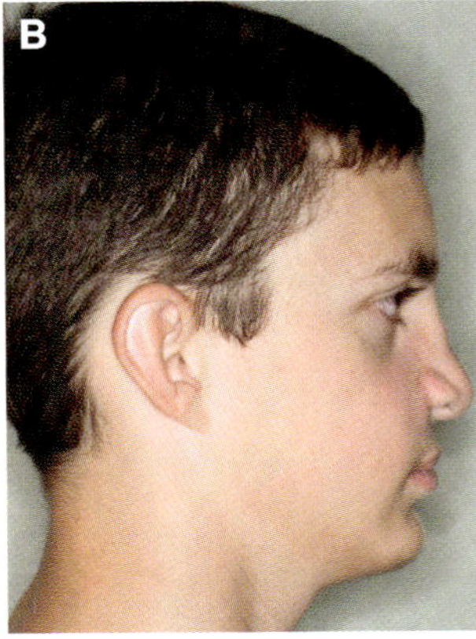

Fig. 21. A comparison of a patient before (*A*) and after (*B*) maxillary distraction. In this patient, distraction includes the amount (15.5 mm) and direction of the advancement as well as the rotation necessary to place the maxilla in an ideal occlusion. (See text relating to this figure on page 13.) (*From*: Yamaji KE, Gateno J, Xia JJ, Teichgraeber JF. New internal Le Fort I distractor for the treatment of midface hypoplasia. J Craniofac Surg. 2004;15(1)124–7.)

computer model to the patient. The transfer of this information is accomplished by creating a surgical template. This template is designed in the computer (Fig. 18a) (Figure 18 located on page 10 of this article.) and fabricated by a stereolithographic apparatus (see Fig. 18b). Fig. 19 (Figure 19 located on page 11 of this article.) shows a comparison of a patient before and after mandibular distraction.

Maxillary distraction

The surgical planning of maxillary distraction is not as complex as in planning for mandibular distraction. In patients with simple maxillary deformities, distraction planning can be accomplished using direct anthropometric measurements, dental models, and cephalometric radiographs. However, in patients with complex maxillary deformities, it is the best to accomplish distraction planning using 3D CASS.

As in planning mandibular distraction, the first step in the maxillary planning process is to reconstruct a 3D computer model of the facial skeleton from a CT scan of the patient's maxillofacial region. This enables visualization and manipulation of the facial skeleton in three dimensions. After the computer model is created, Le Fort I osteotomy is simulated. Using a

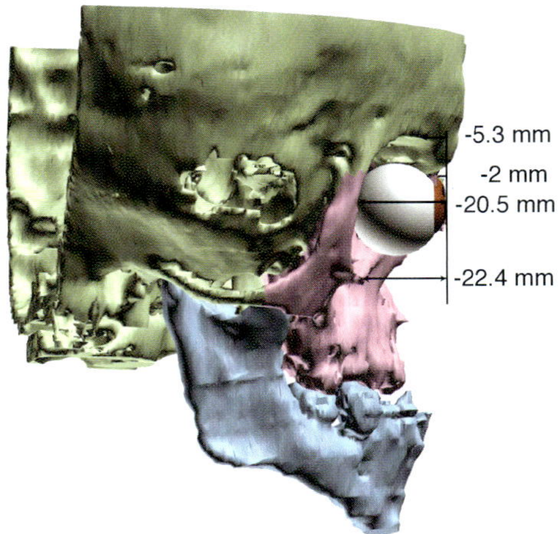

Fig. 22. The magnitude of the midface advancement is determined by the sagittal relationships of the cornea to the supraorbital rim, nasion, lateral rim, and orbitale. (See text relating to this figure on page 14.) (*From*: Gateno J, Teichgraeber JF, Xia JJ. Three-dimensional surgical planning for maxillary and midface distraction osteogenesis. J Craniofac Surg 2003; 14(6):833–9.)

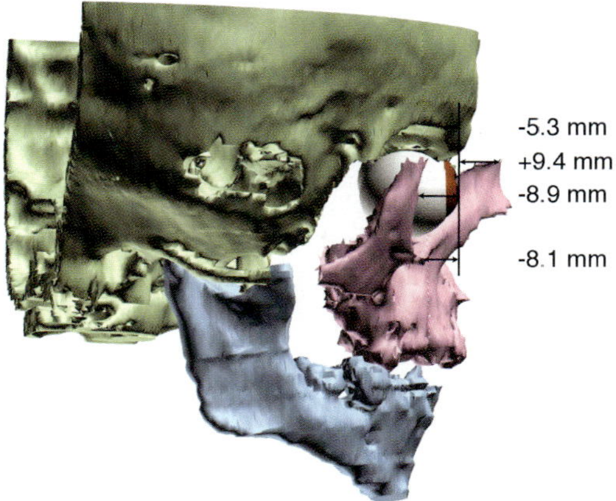

Fig. 23. To simultaneously normalize the occlusion during midface advancement may produce enophthalmos and distortion of the orbitozygomatic region. (See text relating to this figure on page 14.) (*From*: Gateno J, Teichgraeber JF, Xia JJ. Three-dimensional surgical planning for maxillary and midface distraction osteogenesis. J Craniofac Surg 2003;14(6):833–9.)

virtual knife, the maxillary segment is separated from the remaining part of the maxillofacial skeleton.

The next step is to move the segment to the desired final position. A common clinical complication of maxillary distraction is the creation of an anterior open bite, which is produced when the force of distraction is applied below the maxillary center of resistance. The center of resistance is defined as a point at which an applied force produces linear displacement without rotation. If the force is applied below the center of resistance, a counterclockwise rotation will be introduced, resulting in an anterior open-bite (Fig. 20a) (Figure 20 located on page 11 of this article.). This complication can be prevented by applying force above the center of resistance, which will produce a clockwise rotation of the maxilla (see Fig. 20b). Therefore, it is important to calculate the maxillary center of resistance when simulating maxillary distraction. Unfortunately, currently available software is unable to make this calculation. However, the center of mass can be calculated using the modeling software. Up to this point, the authors have assumed that the center of resistance corresponds to the center of mass; the inherent weakness of this assumption is recognized, but clinical results using this assumption have been good.

The final step is to create an animation for the movement of the Le Fort I segment. This animation helps the surgeon visualize the path that the Le Fort segment should take during

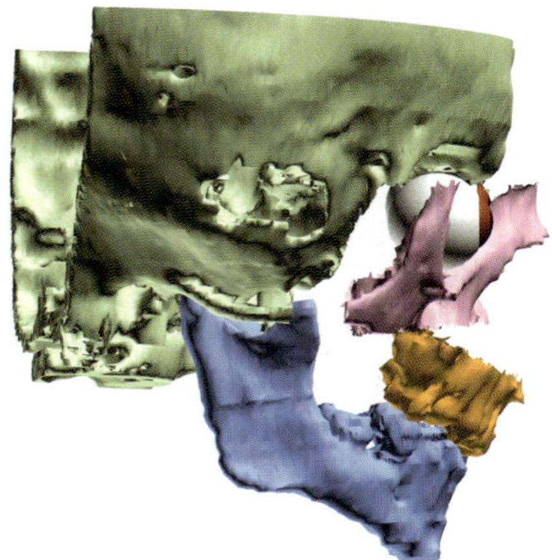

Fig. 24. Normalization of the occlusion is best accomplished by a Le Fort I osteotomy at the completion of facial growth. (See text relating to this figure on page 14.) (*From*: Gateno J, Teichgraeber JF, Xia JJ. Three-dimensional surgical planning for maxillary and midface distraction osteogenesis. J Craniofac Surg 2003;14(6):833–9.)

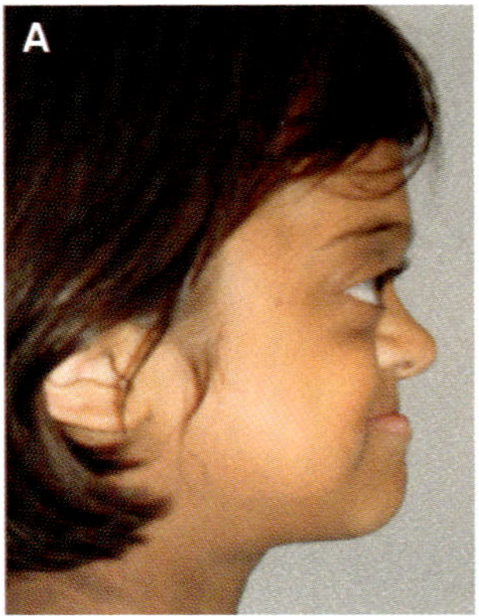

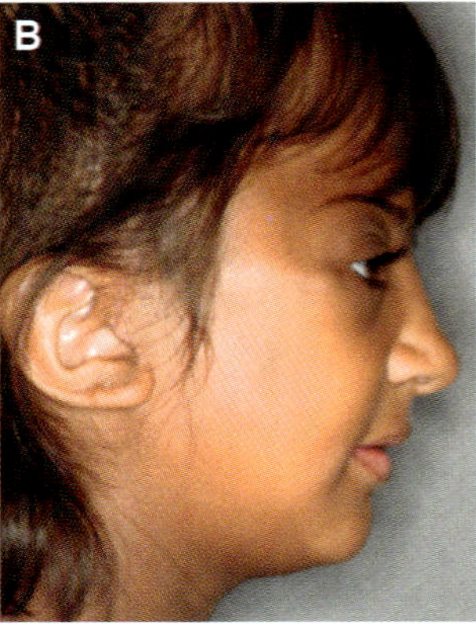

Fig. 25. A comparison of a patient before (*A*) and after (*B*) midface distraction. (See text relating to this figure on page 14.) (*From*: Gateno J, Teichgraeber JF, Xia JJ. Three-dimensional surgical planning for maxillary and midface distraction osteogenesis. J Craniofac Surg 2003;14(6):833–9.)

distraction. The authors have noted that in most patients this path is curvilinear. This curvilinear path is the result of the combination of translation and rotation of the maxilla during distraction. The computer simulation provides the surgeon with a recipe for distraction. Fig. 21 (Figure 21 located on page 12 of this article.) shows a comparison of a patient before and after maxillary distraction. In this patient, distraction includes the amount (15.5 mm) and direction of the advancement as well as the rotation necessary to place the maxilla in ideal occlusion.

Midface distraction

Distraction osteogenesis for monobloc and Le Fort III advancements has been used to treat patients with craniofacial synostosis syndromes. The planning for distraction osteogenesis of the upper face or midface does not differ significantly from the planning of these operations without distraction. Planning always involves a systematic analysis of the deformity and quantification of the deformity in three dimensions. The decision on which surgical approach to use will depend on the patient's midface and anterior cranial base morphology. The major advantage of 3D computer models is that it allows the planner to visualize and adjust the horizontal and vertical relationships in the orbital rims to the globes.

The first step in the planning processes is to build a computerized 3D CT model of the facial skeleton. Additionally, a pair of virtual globes is incorporated into the 3D CT model. The osteotomies are then simulated, and the midface is moved to the desired position. Because the main goal of midface advancement is to normalize the anatomy of the orbitozygomatic region, the magnitude of the anterior advancement is determined by the sagittal relationships of the cornea to the supraorbital rim, nasion, lateral rim, and orbitale (Fig. 22) (Figure 22 located on page 12 of this article.). The use of these relationships helps prevent enophthalmos in patients with midface advancement. A Le Fort III osteotomy is indicated in the treatment of midface hypoplasia if the contour of the forehead and anterior projection of the supraorbital ridge are normal and there is no hypertelorism. A monobloc osteotomy is indicated in midface hypoplasia if there is a decreased anterior projection of the supraorbital ridge and an abnormal contour to the forehead. If orbital hypertelorism is present, a facial bipartition can be completed, and the orbits can be repositioned medially. It is important to keep in mind that the normalization of the vertical and horizontal dimension of the orbital rim takes precedence over the normalization of the occlusion. Any attempt to simultaneously normalize the occlusion may produce enophthalmos and distortion of the orbitozygomatic region (Fig. 23) (Figure 23 located on page 13 of this article.). Normalization of the occlusion is best accomplished by a Le Fort I osteotomy at the completion of facial growth (Fig. 24) (Figure 24 located on page 13 of this article.). Fig. 25 (Figure 25 located on page 14 of this article.) shows a comparison of a patient before and after midface distraction.

Acknowledgments

The authors would like to thank the following people for their help in the project: Ron Kikinis M.D., Professor, Department of Radiology, and Director of Surgical Planning Laboratory, Brigham and Women's Hospital and Harvard Medical School, Boston, MA; Michael A.K. Liebschner Ph.D., Assistant Professor; and Mr. Jeremy J. Lemoine, Graduate Student, Department of Bioengineering, Rice University, Houston, TX; Mr. Andrew M. Christensen, President and Chief Technical Officer of Medical Modeling LLC, Golden, CO.

Suggested readings

Bell WH, editor. Modern practice in orthognathic and reconstructive surgery. Philadelphia: WB Saunders; 1992.

Bell WH, editors. Surgical correction of dentofacial deformities. Philadelphia: WB Saunders; 1980.

Chin M, Toth BA. Le Fort III advancement with gradual distraction using internal devices. Plast Reconstr Surg 1997; 100:819–30 [discussion: 831–2].

Cohen SR. Midface distraction. Semin Orthod 1999;5:52–8.

Ellis E III, Tharanon W, Gambrell K. Accuracy of face-bow transfer: effect on surgical prediction and postsurgical result. J Oral Maxillofac Surg 1992;50:562–7.

Gateno J, Teichgraeber JF, Xia J, inventors. Method and apparatus for fabricating orthognathic surgical splints. US Patent 6,671,539. December 30, 2001.

Gateno J, Teichgraeber JF, Xia JJ. Three-dimensional surgical planning for maxillary and midface distraction osteogenesis. J Craniofac Surg 2003;14:833–9.

Gateno J, Xia J, Teichgraeber JF, et al. A new technique for the creation of a computerized composite skull model. J Oral Maxillofac Surg 2003;61:222–7.

Gateno J, Xia J, Teichgraeber JF, et al. The precision of computer-generated surgical splints. J Oral Maxillofac Surg 2003;61:814–7.

Gosain AK. Distraction osteogenesis of the craniofacial skeleton. Plast Reconstr Surg 2001;107:278–80.

Lambrecht JT. 3D modeling technology in oral and maxillofacial surgery. Chicago: Quintessence; 1995.

Motoki DS, Altobelli DE, Mulliken JB. Enophthalmos following orbital transposition for craniofacial malformations. Plast Reconstr Surg 1993;91:416–22 [discussion: 423–8].

Pai L, Kohout MP, Mulliken JB. Prospective anthropometric analysis of sagittal orbital-globe relationship following fronto-orbital advancement in childhood. Plast Reconstr Surg 1999;103:1341–6.

Papadopoulos MA, Christou PK, Athanasiou AE, et al. Three-dimensional craniofacial reconstruction imaging. Oral Surg Oral Med Oral Pathol Oral Radiol Endod 2002;93:382–93.

Polley JW, Figueroa AA. Management of severe maxillary deficiency in childhood and adolescence through distraction osteogenesis with an external, adjustable, rigid distraction device. J Craniofac Surg 1997;8:181–5 [discussion: 186].

Posnick JC. The craniofacial dysostosis syndromes: current reconstructive strategies. Clin Plast Surg 1994;21:585–98.

Santler G. 3-D COSMOS: a new 3-D model based computerized operation simulation and navigation system. J Maxillofac Surg 2000;28:287–93.

Santler G. The Graz hemisphere splint: a new precise, non-invasive method of replacing the dental arch of 3D-models by plaster models. J Craniomaxillofac Surg 1998;26:169–73.

Toth BA, Kim JW, Chin M, et al. Distraction osteogenesis and its application to the midface and bony orbit in craniosynostosis syndromes. J Craniofac Surg 1998;9:100–13 [discussion: 119–22].

Wong GB, Kakulis EG, Mulliken JB. Analysis of fronto-orbital advancement for Apert, Crouzon, Pfeiffer, and Saethre-Chotzen syndromes. Plast Reconstr Surg 2000;105:2314–23.

Xia J, Ip HH, Samman N, et al. Computer-assisted three-dimensional surgical planning and simulation: 3D virtual osteotomy. Int J Oral Maxillofac Surg 2000;29:11–7.

Xia J, Wang D, Samman N, et al. Computer-assisted three-dimensional surgical planning and simulation: 3D color facial model generation. Int J Oral Maxillofac Surg 2000;29:2–10.

Xia J, Samman N, Yeung RW, et al. Computer-assisted three-dimensional surgical planning and simulation: 3D soft tissue planning and prediction. Int J Oral Maxillofac Surg 2000;29:250–8.

Xia J, Ip HH, Samman N, et al. Three-dimensional virtual-reality surgical planning and soft-tissue prediction for orthognathic surgery. IEEE Trans Inf Technol Biomed 2001;5:97–107.

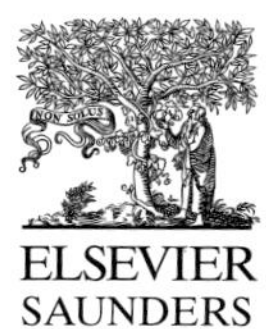
ELSEVIER
SAUNDERS

Atlas Oral Maxillofacial Surg Clin N Am 13 (2005) 41–49

Atlas of the Oral and Maxillofacial Surgery Clinics

Computer-Assisted Navigational Surgery in Oral and Maxillofacial Surgery

Arnulf Baumann, MD, DMD*, Kurt Schicho, DSc, Clemens Klug, MD, Arne Wagner, MD, DMD, Rolf Ewers, MD, DMD

University Hospital of Cranio-Maxillofacial and Oral Surgery, Medical University of Vienna, AKH, Währinger Gürtel 18-20, 1090 Vienna, Austria

The development of computer-assisted navigational surgery has made tremendous progress since the first application of a computer-aided navigation system in a neurosurgical procedure by Watanabe [1] in the late 1980s. Computer-assisted surgery (CAS) is now in widespread use in neurosurgery, orthopedics, and ear, nose, and throat procedures. In oral and maxillofacial surgery, this technique has been applied in dental implantology for the correction of posttraumatic deformities, arthroscopy of the temporomandibular joint, tumor surgery, and removal of foreign bodies.

CAS allows an interactive operative application of CT and MRI scan data, which assists the surgeon during the operative procedure. Therefore, distances and relationships between important anatomic structures can be better evaluated with this technique. Computer-assisted surgery also provides the possibilities of performing less invasive approaches and passing through a preoperative simulated and planned procedure more easily and precisely.

Workflow for navigation procedures

To apply navigational surgery, the patient must first be prepared with reference markers. The markers are necessary for registration of the patient in the navigation system. Reference markers can be inserted in an occlusion splint or as microscrews in the bone. It has been shown that using screws as markers will give the best accuracy. The diagnostic workup by CT or MRI scan is performed with these reference markers in position.

Diagnostic images

Computer-assisted navigational surgery needs CT and MRI scans in high quality. All of the following steps in planning and operative navigation are based on CT and MRI data in three-dimensional (3D) computer models.

Planning and simulation

For simulation and planning, virtual three-dimensional graphics software should be available to allow interactive manipulation, for example in positioning implants according prosthodontic

This work was supported by Grant P-12489 Med from the Austrian Science Foundation (FWF) and by CMF Vienna.

* Corresponding author.

E-mail address: arnulf.baumann@akh-wien.ac.at (A. Baumann).

1061-3315/05/$ - see front matter
doi:10.1016/j.cxom.2004.10.002

requirements. Limitations in the interactive manipulation may require additional planning tools, such as a stereolithographic (SL) model.

Operative procedure

Before starting the operation, the patient must be registered or calibrated using the reference markers (screws or an occlusion splint). Also, the surgical instrument (eg, a drill for implant insertion) must be calibrated relative to the bone. Calibration is performed by sensors attached to the handpiece and to the patient. For this procedure, the optoelectric tracking system with light-emitting diodes is used. The optoelectric tracking system gives better accuracy and stability of the navigation system in comparison with the electromagnetic tracking system, because the magnetic field will be distorted by the motor of the drill.

Two examples explain the current technique and possibilities of computer-assisted navigational surgery in oral and maxillofacial surgery. In these two procedures, the authors used different methods for registration, planning, and intraoperative navigation.

Computer-assisted navigation in posttraumatic zygomatic correction

Posttraumatic malposition of the zygomatic bone may cause flatness of the malar prominence, orbita dystopia with functional symptoms such as diplopia, or a reduced mouth opening. Surgical correction can be performed either by onlay grafts in a matter of camouflage or by an osteotomy of the zygomatic complex. The disadvantage of camouflage is that many symptoms of posttraumatic zygomatic deformity still remain. Therefore, Freihofer and Borstlap [2] and Cohen and Kawamoto [3] suggest a complete osteotomy of the zygomatic bone. However, finding the "right" position of the zygomatic complex to correct facial asymmetry is the most difficult part in the operation because of limited access, even though a coronal approach is used. The change of the anatomic landmarks makes this procedure more difficult than in a "fresh" zygomatic fracture.

The patient presented with several secondary camouflage corrections that had been performed for primary treatment of a right communicated zygomatic fracture. Nevertheless, the patient was not satisfied with the aesthetic outcome (Fig. 1). For the correction procedure, we used a combination of CAS with an SL model, and for the registration procedure we used an occlusion splint with inserted reference markers.

Preoperative planning

Diagnostic data

For planning and simulation of the zygomatic osteotomy, we used an SL model. The SL model was fabricated with the occlusion splint according to the CT data and showed the 3D skeletal structure very precisely. In Fig. 2, different views of the skeletal structure show the lowered right infraorbital rim and the flatness in the right zygomatic prominence.

The SL model was adapted for preoperative treatment planning and also for preoperative registration by using a special occlusion splint. The splint was supplied with marker spheres (at a diameter of 1 mm), and these reference markers were visible in the CT slices. To transfer the marker points to the 3D model, additional horizontal connection bars were added to the surface of the SL model, as seen in Fig. 2. During the production of the SL model, a defined space in the bars was spared, and this space was later filled with 1-mm diameter steel globules (see Fig. 2B). This transfer of the occlusion splint allows registering or calibrating the 3D model in the navigation system.

Surgical planning

According to SL model analysis, the decisions for locating the osteotomy lines were determined, and the surgical procedure was simulated on the SL model. The "right" position of the zygomatic bone was found by comparison with the uninjured side, and the osteotomized segment was fixed with miniplates. These miniplates were later used for fixation of the bone.

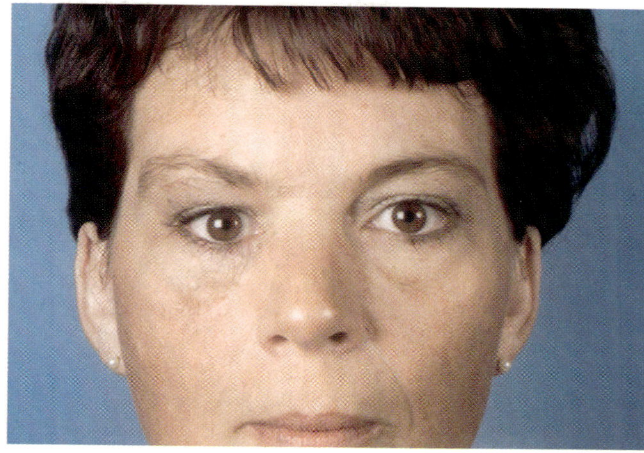

Fig. 1. The patient presented after undergoing several corrections of a right communicated fracture of the zygoma. The right orbit is lowered (orbita dystopia), and the right malar prominence is missing.

Additionally the osteotomy gaps can be visualized directly, which gives the surgeon additional information such as how much bone must be excised for the elevation of the zygomatic complex during the surgery (Fig. 3).

Registration of the SL model

After the surgical planning, the bent miniplates were removed from the model, and the zygomatic was repositioned in its preoperative situation. A sensor was attached to the model for registration in the navigation system. All reference markers were touched consecutively with a pointer, and the corresponding points were touched on the computer screen. After registration of the SL model, the drill holes were recorded with the pointer, and the coordinates were stored in the computer (Fig. 4).

Surgical procedure

Registration of the patient

Registration of the patient in the navigation system was carried out by using reference markers on the occlusion splint (Fig. 5). Then the splint was removed, and the saved coordinates of the drill holes from the SL model were navigated and marked on the patient by the drill. The osteotomy lines were marked.

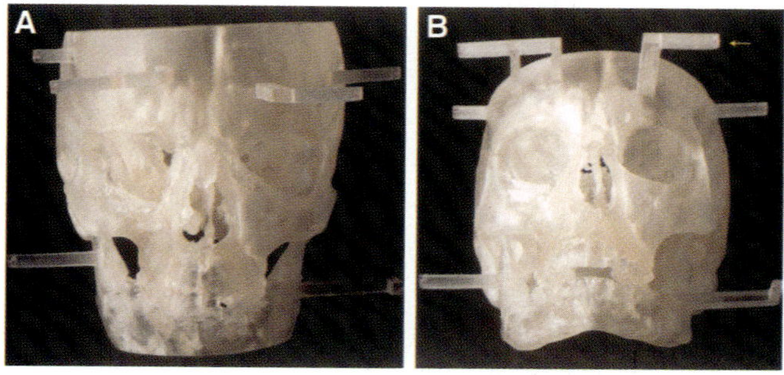

Fig. 2. SL model of the patient in Fig.1. (*A*) Anteroposterior view shows the orbita dystopia and the reconstructed orbital floor. Skeletal asymmetry in the malar prominence can be better seen in the caudal projection (*B*). The arrow (*B*) shows the space for the insertion of the reference markers. These locations correspond to the reference markers in the occlusion splint of the patient.

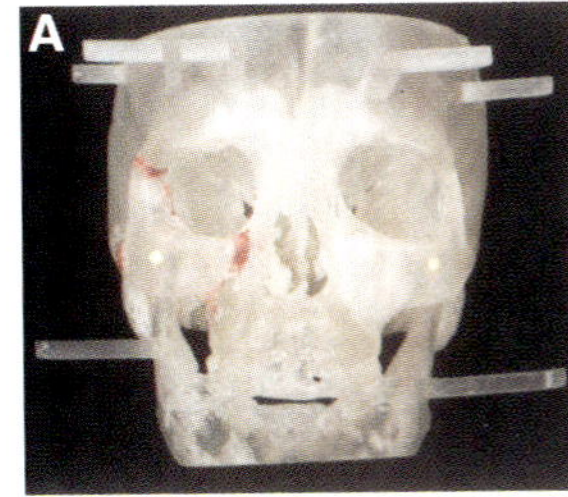

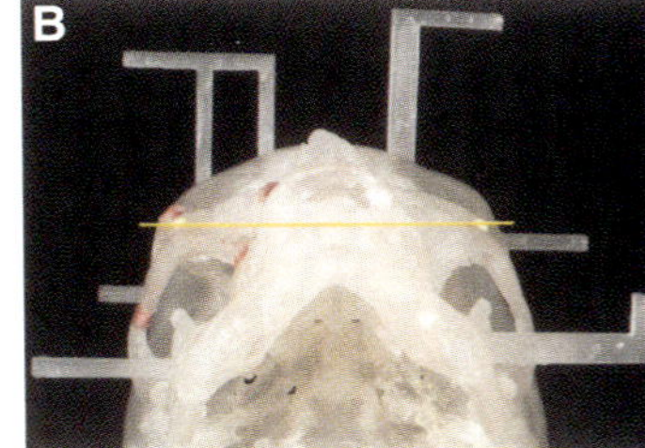

Fig. 3. Postoperative SL model showing anteroposterior (*A*) and caudal (*B*) views. The zygoma was fixed by using miniplates in the "right" position. Miniplates were already removed for sterilization.

Osteotomy

After exposure by buccal, transconjunctival, and lateral eyebrow incisions, the zygomatic bone was osteotomized. Fig. 6 shows the osteotomy at the zygomaticofrontal location and the prepared, navigated drill holes for the osteosynthesis plate. After mobilization, the prebent plates were fixed in the navigated screw holes, and the zygomatic was repositioned according to the curvature of the plate. In addition, orbital floor reconstruction was performed, with a bone graft from the mandible. The clinical outcome resulted in an improvement of the zygomatic position and symmetry in the orbital region (Fig. 7).

Disadvantages of computer-assisted surgery in zygomatic correction

The navigation system is expensive and time consuming, and there are different types of navigation systems available. The authors used the Treon system (Medtronic, Inc, Minneapolis, MN). Marmulla and Niederdellmann [4] used a different navigational system for a similar procedure. They used the Surgical Segment Navigator (SSN) system [Marmulla (inventor); Carl Zeiss, Oberkochen, Germany]. In the SSN system, one frame is fixed at the skull and the other one at the osteotomized zygomatic complex. The osteotomized bone is then navigated to the "right" position. This technique needs more dissection and limits space during zygomatic fixation with miniplates.

Advantages of computer-assisted surgery in zygomatic correction

The planned surgical correction can be better transformed with assistance from the navigation system. CAS may also allow performing a less invasive procedure. The three

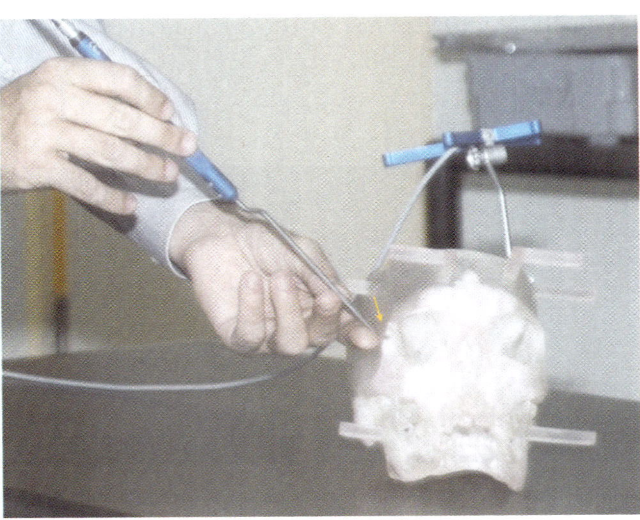

Fig. 4. Registration of the screw holes with the pointer at the SL model. Screw holes are shown at the zygomaticofrontal region (*arrow*).

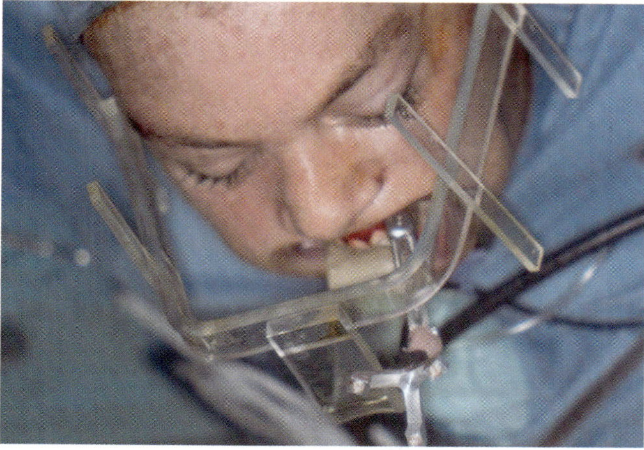

Fig. 5. The patient is registered intraoperatively by using the reference markers on the occlusion splint.

incisions (enoral, transconjunctival, and lateral brow incision) that the present authors used in this case were adequate for performing the osteotomy and finding the "right" position of the zygomatic bone. The prebent plates reduced the operation time. Improvement in 3D software development may shorten preoperative planning time and the navigation procedure itself.

Computer-assisted navigation in dental implantology

Dental implantology may be another application for computer-assisted navigation surgery. The use of presently available commercial software allows for planning the procedure more easily. CAS may help to insert implants more precisely and will provide higher safety against nerve damage or injury of adjacent teeth. A typical workflow for navigated insertion of dental implants in the maxilla is described using a patient case history.

Preoperative planning

Diagnostic data

The CT scan was performed after insertion of microscrews in the maxilla. The screws were used as reference markers for the registration and the navigation (Fig. 8A).

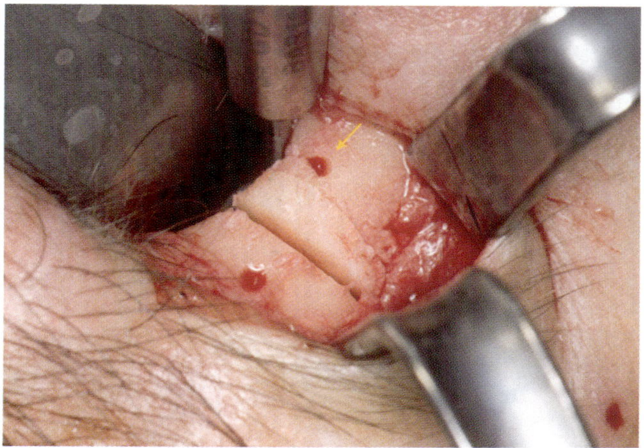

Fig. 6. Intraoperative view of the zygomaticofrontal region. The arrow marks the navigated position of the planned screw position. The bone slice must be removed for the later elevation of the zygoma.

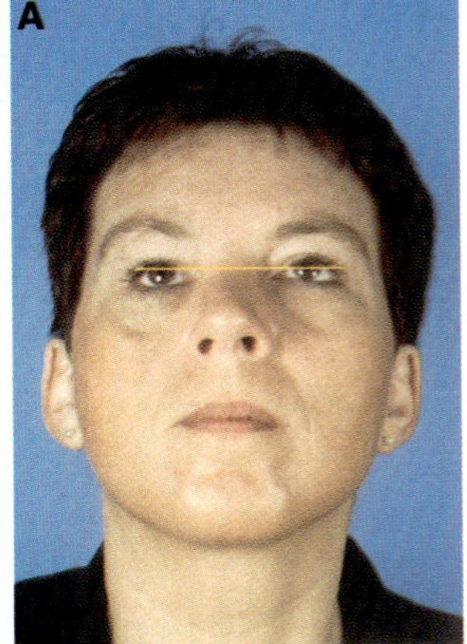

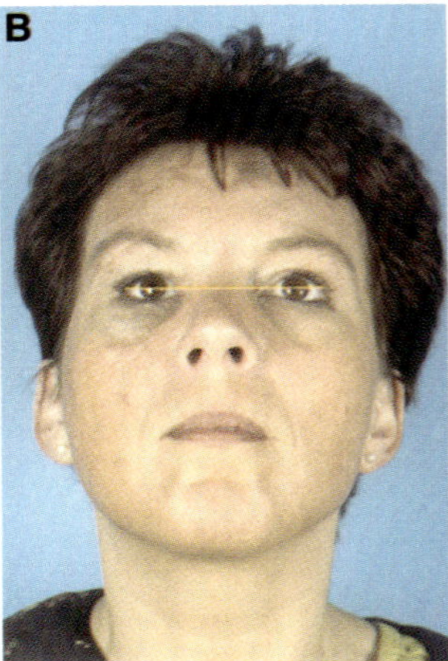

Fig. 7. The caudal view shows the change of the zygoma prominence in the preoperative (*A*) view and after zygoma correction (*B*). The yellow line through the pupil also marks the change of the orbita dystopia.

Planning

After importing the CT data and drawing the dental arc, the implants were positioned according to prosthodontic aspects. For planning and navigation, the authors used the software program of the Virtual Implant System (Artma Medical Technologies AG, Vienna, Austria). This program runs on Apple computers (Apple Inc., Cupertino, California). The implants were selected from a menu on the computer screen and positioned by "drag and drop" using the mouse. In various 2D and 3D renderings, the position, angulations, and lengths of the implants were defined (see Fig. 8B–D). In a case of implantation in the mandible, the alveolar nerve must first be drawn or marked in the CT scan to recognize the various distances to this critical area.

Surgical procedure

Registration of the patient

The patient was registered by markers on the upper jaw. To trace the position of the drill relative to the bone, a navigation sensor was mounted to the patient at the anterior nasal spine, and another sensor was mounted to the handpiece of the drill (Fig. 9).

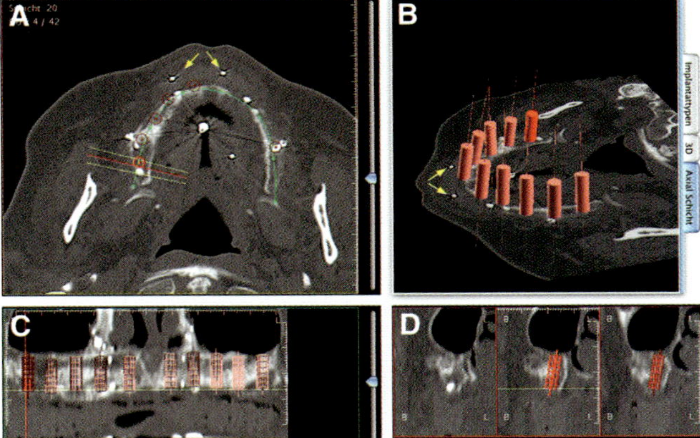

Fig. 8. (*A*) Axial CT scan with inserted screws as reference markers (*arrows*). (*A–D*) Preoperative planning of implant positions and orientation in the maxilla with the Virtual Implant Navigator.

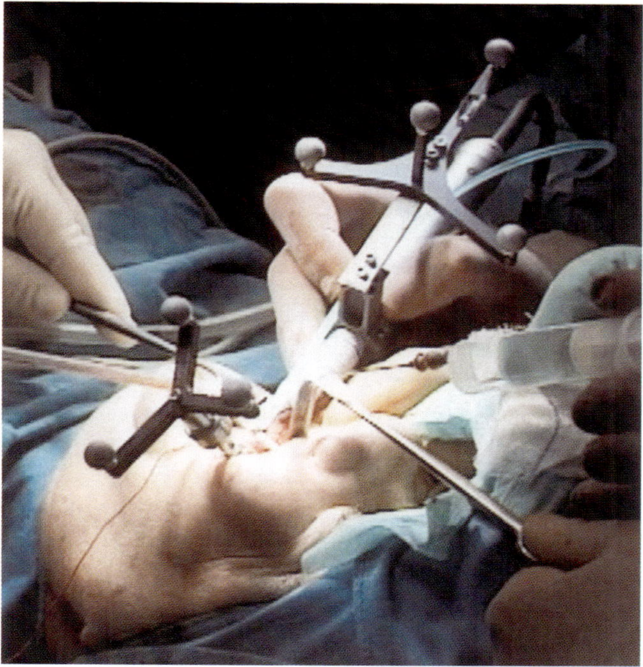

Fig. 9. Operation site. Navigation sensors are attached to the patient and to the handpiece of the dental drill.

Implantation

During the surgical procedure, the actual position of the drill was continuously displayed in relation to the preplanned (optimal) positions of the implants (Fig. 10). The position and angulation of the drill were visible directly on the screen and could be corrected immediately. Fig. 11 shows, for example, the situation in which the drill was in the implant cavity but the angulation and the depth of the drill were not completely correct to the planned situation. Parallelization could be achieved by minimal angulation of the drill.

Clinical outcome

Postoperative CT scans showed a high degree of correspondence between the postoperative implant position and the planned position (Fig. 12) [5].

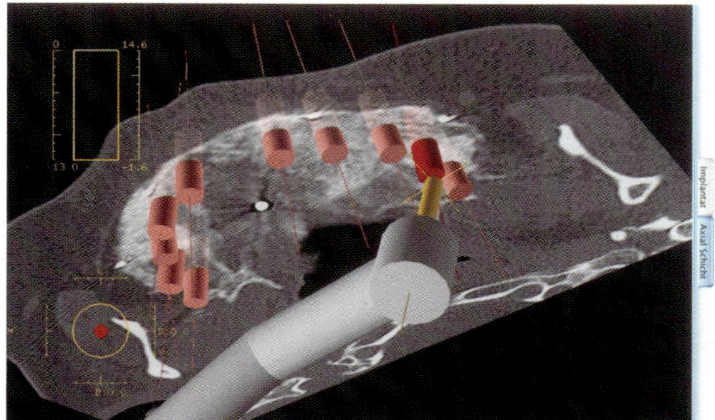

Fig. 10. Position of the drill is shown relative to the preplanned implant position.

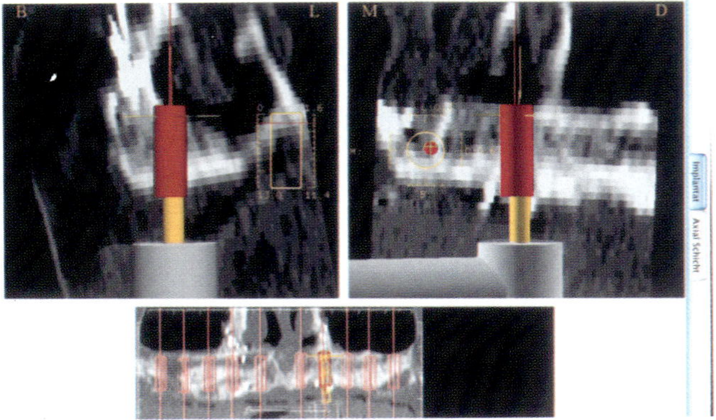

Fig. 11. Intraoperative screens. Various 2D and 3D visualizations are available.

Disadvantages of computer-assisted surgery in dental implantology

The available equipment is expensive, and planning and performing this procedure take more time than a conventional implant insertion procedure. In addition to the Virtual Implant System, the authors also used VISIT (Birkfellner, Center for Biomedical Engineering and Physics, Medical University, Vienna, Austria) software for planning and navigation of the implants [6]. This system runs on the SGI work station (SGI, Mountain View, CA).

Advantages of computer-assisted surgery in dental implantology

Dental implants can be positioned optimally considering functional and prosthodontic aspects. Necessary changes during the surgical procedure can be more easily performed by computer-assisted navigational surgery in comparison with conventional planning with the splint method. Planning changes such as additional or fewer implants or using other implant diameters can be undertaken at any time during the intervention. Also, for the mandible, nerve injury can be avoided, and operative safety is increased.

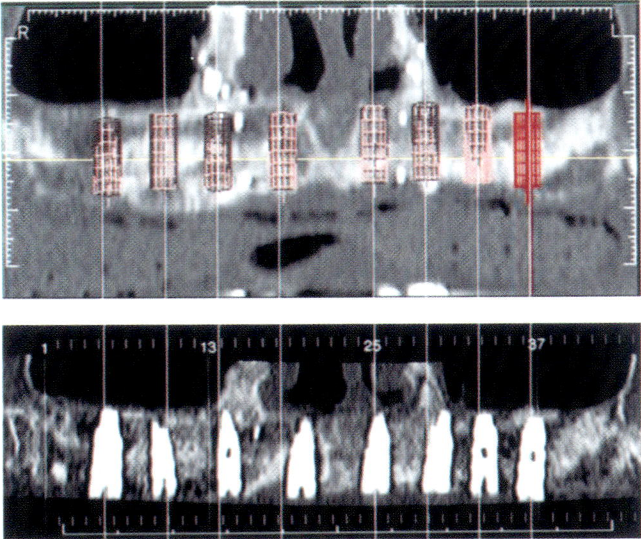

Fig. 12. Comparison of the planned (*top*) and postoperative (*bottom*) implant position in the CT scan. (*From* Ewers R, Schicho K, Truppe M, et al. Computer-aided navigation in dental implantology: 7 years of clinical experience. J Oral Maxillofac Surg 2004;62:329–34; with permission.)

Using navigated implantology, unfavorable mechanical loading may be avoided. Unfavorable mechanical loading can lead to peri-implant bone atrophy and early loss of the implant [7]. Because of the better preoperative planning and precise implant insertion, "bone-demanded" implant insertion can be avoided. In addition to surgical applications, computer navigated surgery also may be useful for teaching demonstrations and for teleconsultation.

Summary

Computer-assisted navigational surgery offers the possibility to translate a preplanned procedure better into the operating room. However the costs for the navigation systems are very high, and the time for preparation for the surgery is longer in comparison with conventional technique. However, the navigation procedure gives more security, particularly in complex cases, and also may result in a better clinical outcome for the patient. Further development of software programs may reduce the preoperative planning time and time spent during the operation.

Further readings

Birkfellner W, Solar P, Gahleitner A, et al. In-vitro assessment of a registration protocol for image guided implant dentistry. Clin Oral Implants Res 2001;12:69–78.

Grunert P, Darabi K, Espinosa J, et al. Computer-aided navigation in neurosurgery. Neurosurg Rev 2003;26:73–99.

Hassfeld S, Mühling J. Computer assisted oral and maxillofacial surgery - a review and assessment of technology. Int J Oral Maxillofac Surg 2001;30:2–13.

Klein M, Hein A, Lueth T, et al. Robot-assisted placement of craniofacial implants. Int J Oral Maxillofac Implants 2003; 18:712–8.

Meyer U, Wiesmann HP, Runte C, et al. Evaluation of accuracy of insertion of dental implants and prosthetic treatment by computer-aided navigation in minipigs. Br J Oral Maxillofac Surg 2003;41:102–8.

Wanschitz F, Birkfellner W, Watzinger F, et al. Evaluation of accuracy of computer-aided intraoperative positioning of endosseous oral implants in the edentulous mandible. Clin Oral Implants Res 2002;13:59–64.

Watzinger F, Wagner A, Enislidis G, et al. Computer aided navigation in secondary reconstruction of posttraumatic deformities of the zygoma. J Craniomaxillofac Surg 1997;25:198–202.

References

[1] Watanabe E, Watanabe T, Manaka S, et al. Three-dimensional digitizer (Neuronavigator): new equipment for computed tomography-guided stereotaxic surgery. Surg Neurol 1987;27:543–7.

[2] Freihofer HPM, Borstlap WA. Reconstruction of the zygomatic area: a comparison between osteotomy and onlay techniques. J Craniomaxillofac Surg 1989;17:243–8.

[3] Cohen SR, Kawamoto HK. Analysis and results of treatment of established posttraumatic facial deformities. Plast Reconstr Surg 1992;90:574–84.

[4] Marmulla R, Niederdellmann H. Surgical planning of computer-assisted reposition osteotomies. Plast Reconstr Surg 1999;104:938–44.

[5] Ewers R, Schicho K, Truppe M, et al. Computer-aided navigation in dental implantology: 7 years of clinical experience. J Oral Maxillofac Surg 2004;62:329–34.

[6] Birkfellner W, Huber K, Larson A, et al. A modular software system for computer-aided surgery and its application in oral implantology. IEEE Trans Med Imaging 2000;19:616–20.

[7] Hobkirk JA, Havthoulas TK. The incidence of mandibular deformation, implant numbers, and loading position on detected forces in abutments supporting fixed implant superstructures. J Prosthet Dent 1998;80:169–74.

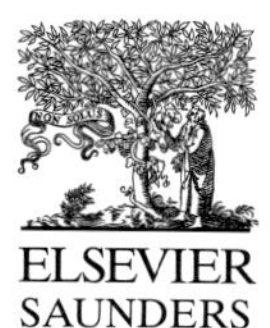
ELSEVIER
SAUNDERS

Atlas Oral Maxillofacial Surg Clin N Am 13 (2005) 51–62

Atlas of the Oral and Maxillofacial Surgery Clinics

Imaging-Guided Biopsy

Hugh D. Curtin, MD[a,b,*], Nina Brogle, MD[c], Paul Caruso, MD[a,b,c]

[a]*Department of Radiology, Harvard Medical School, Boston, MA, USA*
[b]*Department of Radiology, Massachusetts Eye and Ear infirmary, 243 Charles Street Boston, MA 02114, USA*
[c]*Department of Radiology, Massachusetts General Hospital, 55 Fruit Street Boston, MA 02114, USA*

Imaging-guided biopsy allows the sampling of tissue that is not palpable manually or approachable by endoscopy. Imaging identifies the safest approach to a lesion and, during the procedure, confirms the position of the biopsy device relative to the abnormality and to important structures such as the carotid artery. The following article reviews the various techniques used in the head and neck region and emphasizes those techniques that particularly apply in the maxillofacial area.

General considerations

Most biopsies are taken from palpable lesions without image guidance. In the exceptional case where an initial biopsy is not definitive, image guidance can confirm that the sample is indeed from within the questioned abnormality. At the authors' institutions, most candidates for image-guided biopsies have lesions deep to the mandible or in the thyroid region. Thyroid biopsies, which are usually performed with ultrasonography, are beyond the scope of this article.

Primary lesions deep to the mandible can be categorized by their location. The information from initial imaging may obviate the need for definitive preoperative biopsy. However, in many cases, confirmation of histology is requested before planning the definitive therapy. Almost always, imaging can place a lesion into pre- or poststyloid parapharyngeal space, the masticator space, or the retropharyngeal space. Such localization narrows the possible diagnoses into limited categories and may give enough information for planning therapy.

Lesions of the poststyloid parapharyngeal space are typically posterior to the carotid artery. Most are paragangliomas (glomus vagale) or nerve sheath lesions. Although there have been fine needle aspirations of paragangliomas, most clinicians consider the diagnosis established by either imaging (CT or MRI) or occasionally by angiography. Treatment planning does not require biopsy. Similarly, a surgeon may plan a surgical approach or choose long-term monitoring for those less vascular lesions that have no aggressive features and are likely nerve sheath tumors. In the rare case that is not typical of paraganglioma or nerve sheath tumor, an image-guided biopsy may be considered. For instance, an irregular infiltrating margin is not typical of nerve sheath tumors or paraganglioma, and such a lesion is appropriate for biopsy; however, such tumors are extremely rare in the poststyloid space.

Prestyloid lesions pass anterior to the carotid artery and styloid process and posterior to the medial pterygoid muscle and mandibular ramus. Almost all of these lesions are of parotid origin, and most are benign. Most clinicians consider fine needle aspiration a safe procedure, and there are reports of core biopsies performed without complication. Seeding along a needle tract is a theoretical possibility, but documented reports are extremely rare. If a lesion has the

* Corresponding author. Department of Radiology, Massachusetts Eye and Ear infirmary, 243 Charles Street Boston, MA 02114.

E-mail address: hdcurtin@meei.harvard.edu (H.D. Curtin).

1061-3315/05/$ - see front matter
doi:10.1016/j.cxom.2004.10.003

typical appearance of a pleomorphic adenoma without irregular margins or evidence of aggressiveness, some surgeons advise excisional biopsy, preferring to avoid tumor manipulation before a definitive resection.

Tumors medial to the carotid artery usually arise from the sympathetic chain or represent retropharyngeal nodes (nodes of Rouviere). If the lesion is a metastatic node, the primary tumor is usually obvious. Lymphoproliferative lesions usually have other nodes from which biopsies may be obtained more easily. Isolated primary lesions do arise from the sympathetic chain. A biopsy may be considered, but again, imaging may give enough information to establish a clinical plan. The authors commonly perform a biopsy in this area to establish that there is recurrent carcinoma in a node of a patient who has undergone therapy for pharyngeal malignancy.

Masticator space lesions commonly arise from the jaw (osseous or odontogenic tumors) or from the third division of the trigeminal nerve. Mesenchymal tumors are rare. Oral cavity or pharyngeal malignancies can recur here. Preoperative needle aspirations or core biopsies may not be necessary in many mandibular tumors but are frequently helpful for soft tissue lesions.

Techniques

Image-guided biopsies can be performed with an aspiration or a core technique. An attempt may be made to achieve an adequate aspiration, but if this is not achieved, a core is taken. Potential injury to key vessels and nerves is the major concern with a core biopsy.

Aspiration

Thin needles, 20 to 25 gauge, are used for aspirations. Although a simple needle may be chosen, many practitioners prefer a spinal needle, removing the stylet only when the needle is close to or within the lesion. This variation prevents normal tissue from being accidentally pushed into the lumen as the needle approaches the lesion. The presence of the stylet also prevents blood from entering the lumen and clotting in the needle during the delay for scanning to verify position. Most frequently, the authors use a 22, 23 or 25-gauge spinal needle, either 1.5 or 3.5 in long, depending on the depth of the lesion. For CT guidance and position verification, a plastic hub gives much less artifact than a metal one. Some radiologists initially place an 18 or 19-gauge needle close to the lesion. This allows multiple passes with a 23-gauge needle without the need to go through the superficial tissues more than once.

The aspiration technique pulls tissue and fluid from the lesion into the needle or syringe, and hopefully there are enough cells to use cytologic techniques to make a diagnosis. Ideally, the cytotechnologist and pathologist are present during the procedure to evaluate the aspirate and to determine whether sufficient material is present to make the appropriate analysis.

The needle attaches to a syringe directly or connects to the syringe by a short length of tubing. The use of tubing allows the application of suction with less awkward hand position. Some practitioners use a syringe holder to perform the biopsy. As the needle passes into the lesion, a rapid in-and-out sampling motion is combined with gentle twisting in an attempt to pull cellular material into the needle. If fluid, blood, or debris appears in the hub of the syringe, suction is released, and the needle removed. If there is significant blood, the radiologist can make an additional needle pass without suction to minimize the chance of blood passing into the needle.

The sample is squirted onto a slide and smeared for rapid stain. The needle is rinsed with saline, and the irrigation is saved in a tube to be spun down for cell block analysis if the aspirate is not definitive. If there is a question of infection, there is usually more fluid or aspirated material, and this can undergo appropriate stain and cultures.

The best samples may be from the periphery of lesions with significant necrosis. The radiologist may pass the needle into and out of the margin of a lesion to take advantage of the more cellular material or may attempt to pass the needle along the edge of a lesion.

Local anesthesia is usually sufficient for most biopsies. Some radiologists use intravenous pain medication or even some degree of sedation for deeper biopsies. General anesthesia may be required, particularly in children.

The accuracy of aspiration cytology is excellent if there is an adequate sample. An insufficient sample can be a problem, and multiple passes are frequently required; this can be difficult in deeper lesions where passing the needle to the edge of the mass may not be a trivial exercise. In addition, with deeper lesions, the prediction of adequate needle tip movement is more difficult because tissues between the skin and the lesion may compress so that the excursion of the needle within the lesions may be less than that suggested by the movement at the skin surface. The needle may push the lesion rather than penetrate it for an adequate sample. Again, placing an introducer and passing a thinner needle through the larger one gives a coaxial system that may be helpful because there is little resistance within the introducer needle itself.

Core techniques

In core sampling techniques, the designed procedure takes a piece of the tissue or a core through the lesion. Core techniques can use a needle or a specialized biopsy gun. The collected sample goes to pathology for a standard tissue analysis.

There are many core techniques available. A simple larger bore needle can cut out a small piece. Specially designed core biopsy needles have cutting points or point edges to facilitate retrieving small bits of tumor for the sample. Biopsy guns have many designs. For instance, one coaxial system uses a central sampling needle passed through a slightly larger cutting needle (Fig. 1). There is a notch or groove just proximal to the point of the sampling needle that allows tissue to collapse against the needle. The outer needle snaps over the sampling needle, cutting off the tissue that has collapsed against the notch of the inner needle. Because of the size of the needle, multiple complete passes from the surface of the skin may not be practical. Again, an introducer sheath is initially placed, and the actual biopsies are taken with a coaxial needle or gun placed through this outer sheath. Moving the outer sheath slightly between passes allows sampling of different parts of the tumor.

Some systems use a technique in which the point is placed at the edge of the lesion, and the gun fires directly into the abnormality with an in-and-out motion to collect the sample. Other systems allow the practitioner to advance the sampling needle into the lesion manually. This allows the radiologist to feel the consistency as the point advances to the limit of the sample site. The length of the sampling needle and thus the penetration can usually be adjusted. This can be helpful with deeper lesions close to bone where space is limited.

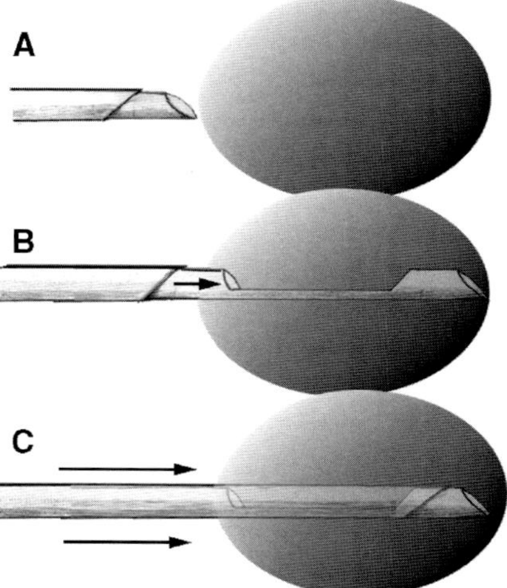

Fig. 1. Core biopsy. (*A*) The coaxial device is passed to the edge of the lesion. (*B*) The inner biopsy needle is then advanced into the lesion. This part of the apparatus contains a notch into which the tissue collapses. (*C*) Finally, the outer cutting sheath snaps over the inner needle, trapping the tissue in the notch of the biopsy inner needle.

Pretesting

Some radiologists pretest patients for various bleeding and clotting parameters before a biopsy procedure; some do not require testing if an aspiration biopsy is planned in a patient who has no history of abnormal bleeding or if the lesion is relatively superficial, where pressure can easily be applied. These authors test patients when a core biopsy is planned or if there is any question of abnormal bleeding in the past. The patient is kept in the department for approximately 1 hour to ensure that there is no significant swelling.

Imaging modalities

Ultrasound, CT, and MRI are useful for guiding the needle placement. Each modality has advantages and disadvantages. The primary considerations include the abilities to visualize the lesion, to predict the position of important structures the operator wishes to avoid, and to visualize movements of the needle in "real time" or by repeat imaging. Real time refers to the ability to visualize the structures as the needle is actually being moved, avoiding the necessity to stop and take an image. Finally, with CT, radiation is a consideration.

Ultrasonography

Ultrasonography is the image guidance form that is probably most easily used, particularly in the neck below the level of the jaw (Fig. 2). This is a real time technique, and specialized biopsy devices allow visualization of the point of the needle during placement. There is no radiation, and the positions of vessels are obvious. Ultrasonography cannot pass through bone or air. The mandible reflects the sound, so areas in the parapharyngeal region are not easily visualized; this is a major problem above the level of the angle of the mandible.

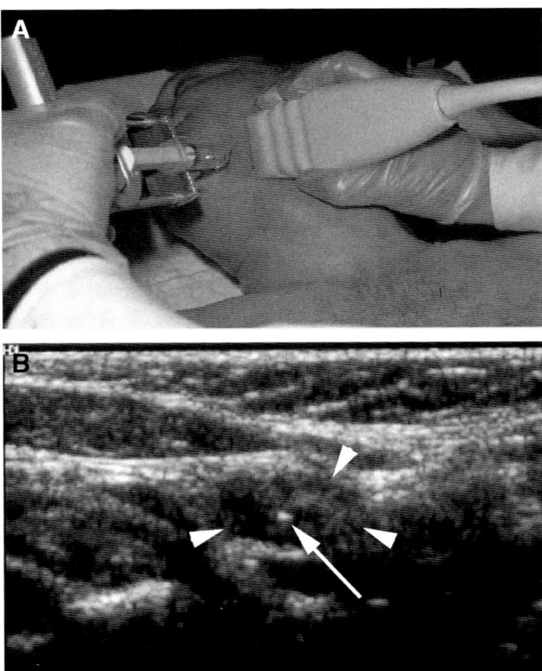

Fig. 2. Ultrasound-guided aspiration of a cervical lymph node. (*A*) Holding the transducer in the right hand, the operator passes the needle into the node. The syringe is held in an apparatus that gives stability and ease of suction application. (*From* Castelijns JA, van den Brekel MWM, et al. Ultrasound of the neck. In: Som PM, Curtin HD, editors. Head and neck imaging. 4th Edition. St. Louis: Mosby; 2003. p. 1936; with permission.) (*B*) The ultrasonography image shows low reflectivity within the node (*arrowheads*). The needle tip is identified by its higher reflectivity (*long arrow*).

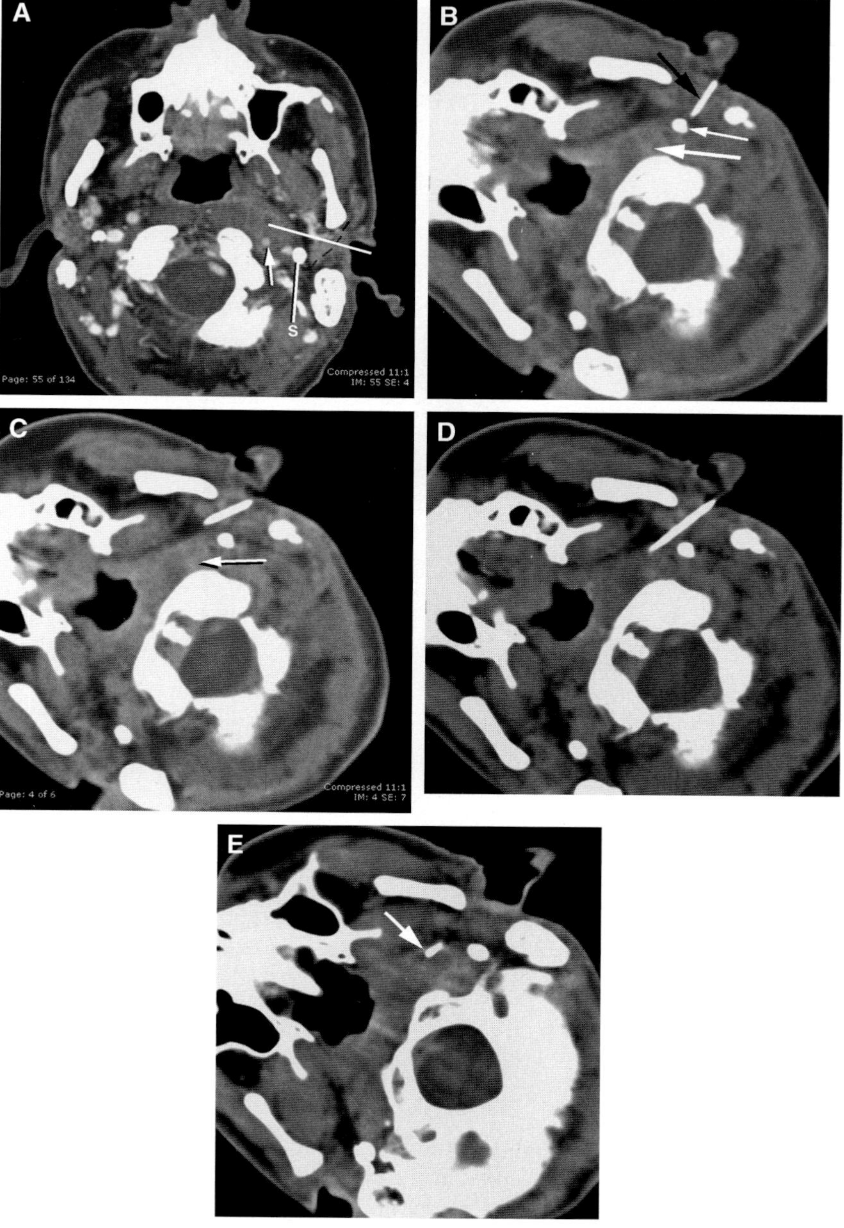

Fig. 3. CT biopsy of a recurrent squamous cell cancer in a node of Rouviere through stylomandibular tunnel. (*A*) Initial CT scan identifies the lesion and the carotid artery (*arrow*). The appropriate path to the lesion is indicated by the *white line*. Because this ideal path would pass through the auricle, a slightly anterior approach would be used, or the ear would be pulled slightly forward. S, styloid process; *dotted line*, approximate position and course of the facial nerve. (*B*) The patient is rotated into a lateral oblique position. The carotid artery is no longer visible because the contrast has faded, but the position of the artery can be estimated (*large arrow*) by comparison with the previous contrast-enhanced scan. The styloid process (*small arrow*) is a landmark used to avoid puncturing the carotid. The initial needle used for local anesthesia (*black arrow*) remains in place for an initial approximation of the puncture site. (*C*) The biopsy needle is then passed beyond the plane of the stylomandibular tunnel. At this point, the needle tip is beyond the position of the facial nerve (the *white arrow* approximates the position of the carotid artery). (*D*) The needle tip is advanced to the edge of the lesion. The needle tip is just anterior to the position of the carotid artery. (*E*) The tip of the needle (*arrow*) is within the lesion, and the biopsy sample is taken at this point.

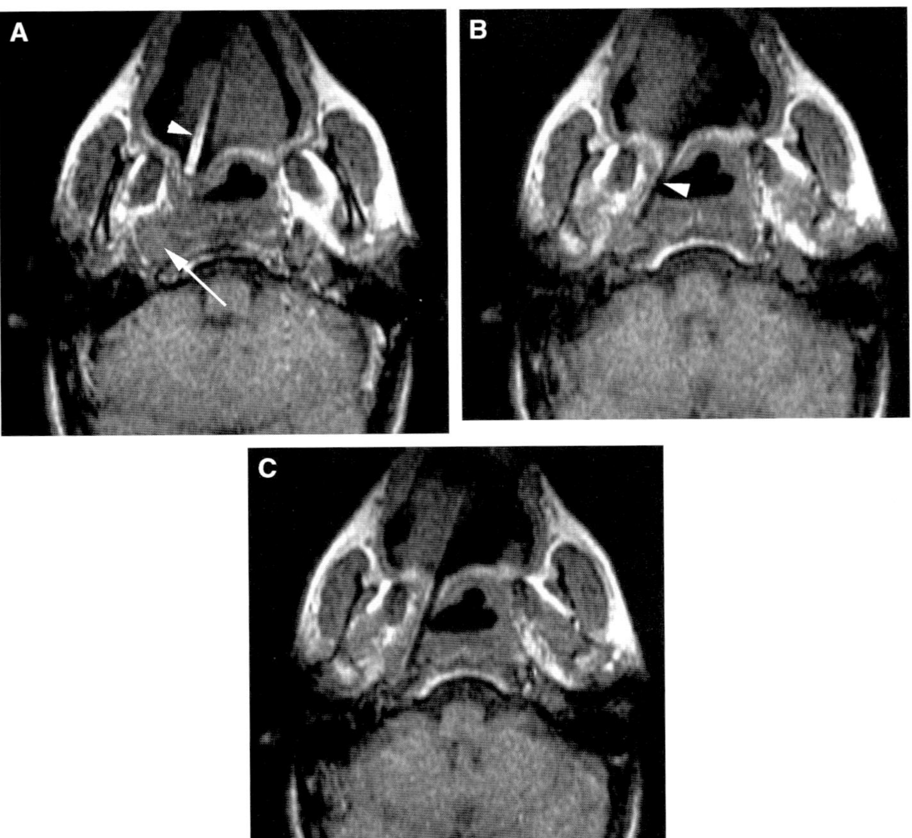

Fig. 4. MRI-guided biopsy of a node of Rouviere (squamous cell carcinoma) performed during real time imaging in an open magnet. The needle position is under constant control of the operator who is in the room during the entire procedure. (*A*) The marker (*arrowhead*) is placed adjacent to the soft palate so that the pathway to the lesion (*arrow*) can be approximated. (*B,C*) A needle (*arrowhead*) is advanced into the abnormality under MRI guidance. The needle tip is visible within the node. (*Courtesy of* Liangge Hsu, MD, Dept. of Radiology, Brigham and Women's Hospital, Harvard Medical School, Boston, MA.)

CT

CT scanning is widely used for areas deep to the mandible, particularly in the parapharyngeal region. CT machines are readily available, and no special instrumentation is required. CT uses ionizing radiation. Careful planning helps to limit the number of required needle position checks. Some CT scanners have a biopsy mode that produces almost a fluoroscopic real time image, but this mode gives a relatively higher dosage of radiation.

A grid that is visible with CT can be placed on the skin over the lesion. Several types of grids are commercially available, but a simple tube or even small drops of barium can be used. CT scanners use a laser to define the vertical (craniocaudal) position of every slice, so the appropriate position of the needle placement is determined by cross-referencing the markers with the laser localizer. In the neck or deep to the mandible, there are usually enough surface landmarks such as the angle of the mandible, the ear, or even a skin crease that are identifiable on the scan so that markers are not necessary.

The authors usually begin with a contrast-enhanced scan through the entire neck, allowing the localization of major vessels and the approximate position of major nerves (Fig. 3). The initial scan can be performed in the neutral position, with the patient in the supine position or in the position of the planned biopsy.

Once the radiologist has defined the location of the artery and the lesion as well as other landmarks, the procedure begins with injection of local anesthetic into the skin. After a slightly deeper injection, the syringe is removed from the needle, leaving the needle in place as a marker.

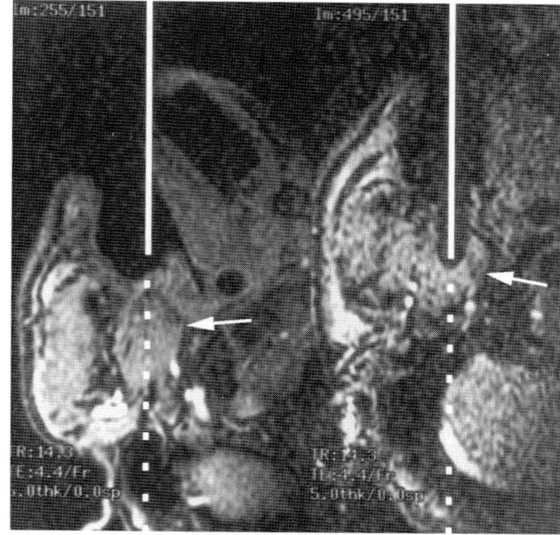

Fig. 5. MRI-guided biopsy of recurrent squamous cell carcinoma in the masticator space. On these two images, a needle can be followed into the site of the lesion (*arrows*) in the region of the medial pterygoid muscle. White line indicates position of the needle. Dotted line indicates trajectory of needle. (*Courtesy of* Liangge Hsu, MD, Dept of Radiology, Brigham and Women's Hospital, Harvard Medical School, Boston, MA.)

A scan is performed through the level of the needle. At this point the contrast has passed, and the carotid artery position must be predicted based on the appearance of the initial CT scan (see Fig. 3B). The biopsy needle is inserted either along the course of the anesthetic needle or in a course that has changed based on the position seen on the scan. The biopsy needle is then advanced toward the lesion. One or two checks using repeat CT scans assure the continued appropriate progress toward the site of interest. With the tip of the needle at the edge of the lesion, either the aspiration is performed or a core biopsy is taken. The cytologist or pathologist confirms the adequacy of an aspirated sample. If a small piece of tissue is obtained by a core technique, the tissue is sent to the pathology department. Time spent on CT scanners is expensive, and biopsies tend to be relatively time intensive.

MRI

MRI-guided biopsies require special equipment. Open machines allow access to the patient during the procedure. Specialized needles designed specifically for MRI-guided procedures are not ferromagnetic and are therefore compatible with use in high magnetic fields in which the use of normal needles is impossible.

MRI does not use ionizing radiation, so there is no concern about obtaining multiple images to verify the position of a needle. The scanners have sequences that allow real time visualization as the needle passes through the tissues into the lesion (Figs. 4, 5). MRI is very expensive, and appropriate "interventional" machines are not widely available. Cases requiring anesthesia need specialized nonferromagnetic anesthesia machines as well.

Approaches and needle placement

There are many approaches available by which a needle or biopsy device may be safely placed in a lesion (Fig. 6). The authors have passed many needles through the region of the facial nerve without facial weakness, although most have been relatively slim needles. Passing needles through the carotid artery is avoided, but they probably have gone through the external carotid artery and many different veins. One could argue that a narrow gauge needle will not cause a problem even with the carotid artery, but because the carotid artery cannot be compressed deep to the mandible and it is relatively easy to avoid, the authors plan needle placement to avoid the vessel.

If one is using a cutting needle or performing a core biopsy, avoiding even medium size vessels, and particularly nerves, is prudent. The authors plan the approach to avoid major nerves, and before taking a core biopsy, the approach ensures that the projected trajectory does not include the path of any major nerve or vessel.

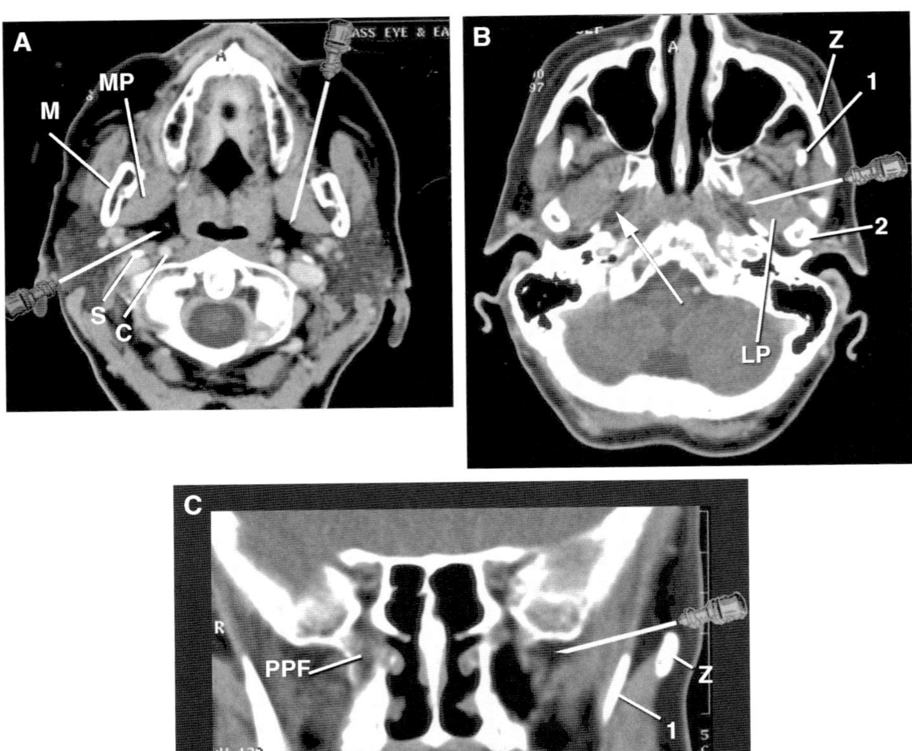

Fig. 6. Approaches. (*A*) Trans-stylomandibular foramen and retromaxillary approaches. Axial CT image at the level of the parotid gland. In the stylomandibular approach (*left*), the needle passes just anterior to the styloid (S) and just posterior to the mandible (M). The needle reaches the parapharyngeal fat, passing just posterior to the internal maxillary artery and retromandibular vein. The styloid process "protects" the carotid artery (C). In the retromaxillary approach (*right*), the needle passes between the maxilla and the mandible. Important structures in this area include the parotid duct. MP, medial pterygoid. (*B*) Transmandibular notch approach. The needle (*right*) passes beneath the zygomatic arch (Z) between the condyle (2) and the coronoid process (1). The needle passes through the mandibular (sigmoid) notch. The position of the third division of trigeminal nerve (V_3) is shown (*arrow*). LP, lateral pterygoid muscle. (*C*) Suprazygomatic approach. The needle passes over the zygomatic arch (Z) and downward into the pterygopalatine fossa. This angle avoids extension of the needle into the orbit. 1, coronoid process; PPF, pterygopalatine fossa on the normal opposite side.

In the lower neck, the pathway is usually straightforward, and the needle passes from the skin directly into the lesion. Most of these biopsies can be performed easily with ultrasonography. The position of the carotid artery and major nerves such as the recurrent laryngeal, phrenic, vagus, and other nerves are constant enough and may at times actually be visible.

CT is usually used for biopsies performed on lesions deep to the mandible in the retropharyngeal and parapharyngeal and medial masticator spaces, and the approaches depend on the position of the lesion. The stylomandibular tunnel, mandibular notch, and intraoral approaches are used as well as the retromaxillary approach through the cheek, angling posteriorly along the medial surface of the mandibular ramus. The pterygopalatine fossa can be approached by passing just over the zygomatic arch. The authors emphasize the stylomandibular approach because this is the approach most commonly used at our institutions, but other approaches will be described briefly as well.

Stylomandibular tunnel

The authors use the stylomandibular tunnel for most biopsies deep to the mandible. In these authors' experience, this is very well tolerated, and only local anesthetic has been used for the procedure (Figs. 7, 8) (see also Fig. 3). Landmarks such as the ear lobe and the mandible ramus allow prediction of the appropriate position for initial skin puncture.

The initial contrast-enhanced scan localizes the lesion and shows the relationship of the carotid artery to the lesion and to the styloid process. This step is unnecessary if a recent CT or MRI has been acquired that adequately shows the relationships. The styloid process has been found to be a useful landmark. The angle chosen to pass the styloid process can render impossible inadvertent penetration of the carotid artery. Even if a biopsy is performed on a node of Rouviere on the far side (medial to) the carotid artery, the lesion usually extends sufficiently

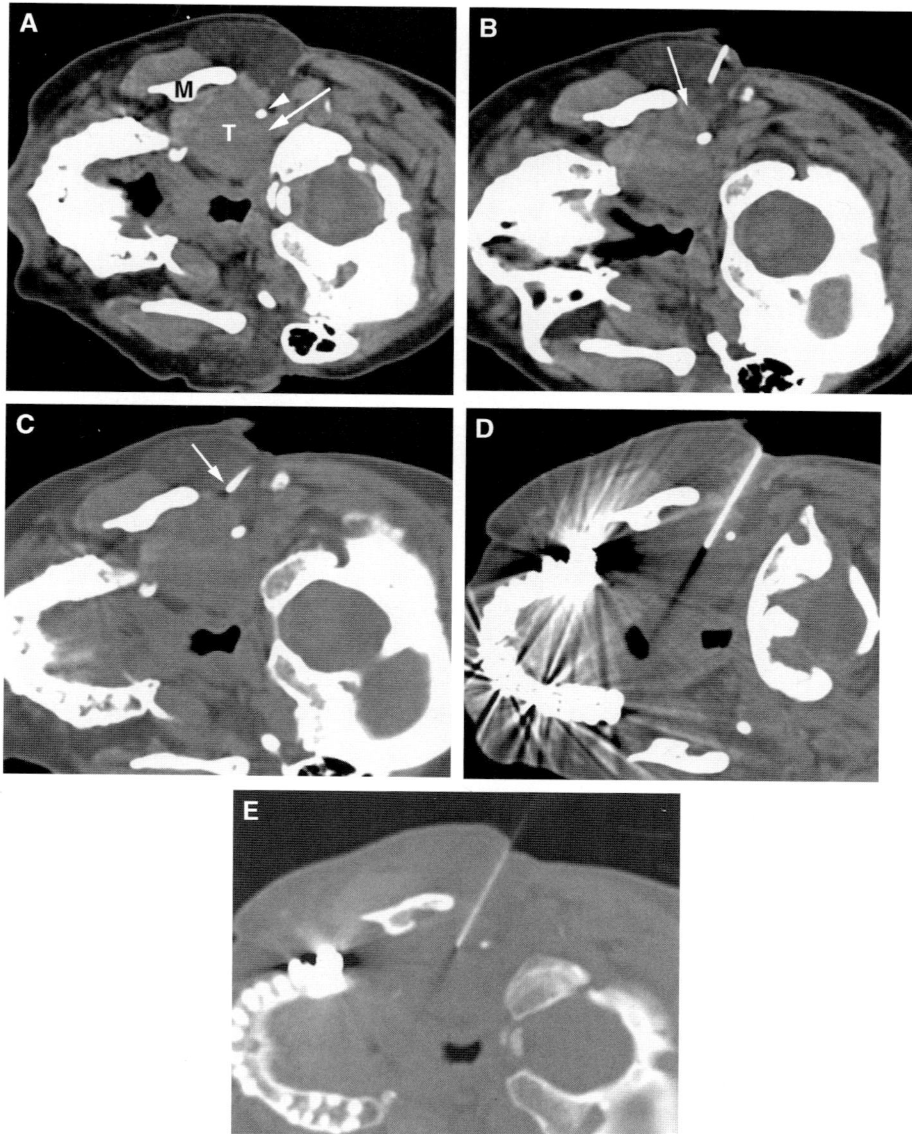

Fig. 7. CT-guided biopsy of pleomorphic adenoma in the prestyloid parapharyngeal space via the stylomandibular tunnel. (*A*) The tumor (T) is visible in the parapharyngeal space. The position of the carotid artery is not visible because this is a noncontrast-enhanced scan, but its position (*arrow*) had been determined on the prebiopsy MRI. The styloid process (*arrowhead*) is the key landmark. M, mandible. (*B*) The needle used for initial local anesthesia is visible in the region of the parotid. The edge of the lesion (*arrow*) bulges through the stylomandibular tunnel. At this point, the lesion cannot be differentiated from the retromandibular vein. (*C*) The anesthesia needle has been replaced by the aspiration cytology needle. The tip of the needle (*arrow*) is now quite close to the plane of the facial nerve. (*D*) The aspiration needle has been passed well beyond the plane of the stylomandibular tunnel into the center of the lesion. If there is significant artifact from dental restoration, the patient tilts the chin upward or downward to change the projected plane for better visualization, as in (*E*). (*E*) Wider window shows the position of the needle.

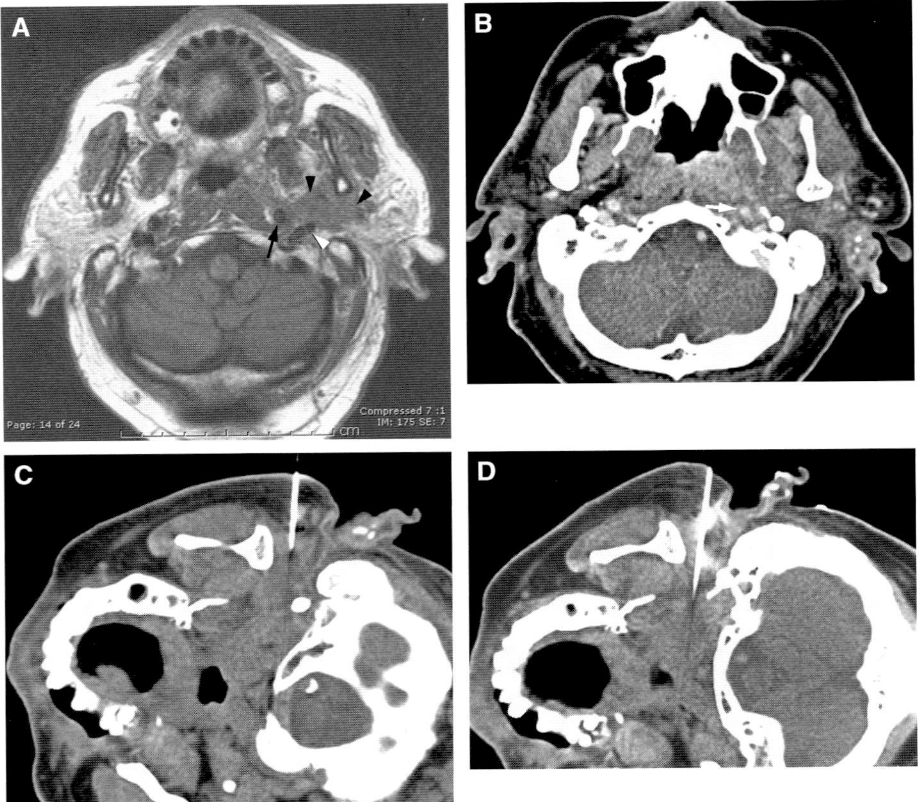

Fig. 8. Core biopsy of the parapharyngeal region. Patient had facial paralysis at the time of presentation. (*A*) MRI shows the lateral part of the lesion (*arrowheads*) in the stylomandibular tunnel, extending into the parapharyngeal space. Images followed more superiorly showed this infiltrative lesion extending to the skull base. Several CT-guided needle aspiration procedures were unsuccessful, as was an endoscopic biopsy performed through the nasopharynx. The carotid artery (*arrow*) and the styloid process (*white arrowhead*) are identified. (*B*) Before needle insertion, a CT scan with contrast confirms the position of the carotid artery (*arrow*). The fascial planes in the parapharyngeal area are obliterated by the process. (*C*) The introducer is passed toward the styloid process. (*D*) Once the introducer is beyond the styloid process, the biopsy needle is passed into the lesion. The carotid artery is not visible, but its position is predictable based on the bony anatomy in the region of the styloid process.

anteriorly so that a safe passage is possible. Occasionally the carotid artery loops forward, making avoidance of the artery more difficult.

The facial nerve exits the stylomastoid foramen and then curves slightly laterally to reach the lateral aspect of the retromandibular vein (see Fig. 3). Core biopsy approaches should avoid this line. The authors have passed the tip of biopsy guns or core needles beyond the plane and taken samples in the deeper regions but do not take biopsies directly from that plane. Aspirations have been performed with multiple passes through this region. An aspiration is preferred rather than a core biopsy if the imaging suggests strongly that a lesion is a pleomorphic adenoma, and the clinician requests verification.

The authors have used this approach for deep retropharyngeal lesions, parapharyngeal tumors, and even masses along the medial cortex of the mandibular ramus. The angle of approach is rotated to achieve access to the various structures.

Mandibular (sigmoid) notch

The mandibular notch gives access to the medial masticator space and to the parapharyngeal and retropharyngeal spaces. Opening the mouth slightly widens the space between the zygomatic arch and the mandibular notch. This approach can avoid a tortuous carotid artery that is unavoidable through the stylomandibular tunnel.

In the authors' experience, this approach is less well tolerated than the stylomandibular approach. The third division of the trigeminal nerve lies just deep to the notch. Exiting the foramen ovale, the nerve passes along the medial aspect of the lateral pterygoid muscle before curving laterally toward the mandibular ramus. The fascial layers and ligaments can be difficult to traverse.

Retromaxillary

Some practitioners prefer passing a needle through the cheek and along the medial surface of the mandible. The mandible ramus is palpable, aiding initial needle positioning. By using the appropriate angle, the carotid is avoidable. Complications relative to the parotid duct have not been reported, but a salivary fistula is a potential complication.

Other approaches

In addition to those approaches discussed, the authors have rarely used a transoral approach and occasionally an approach extending superiorly from beneath the angle of the mandible. The submandibular approach does not allow visualization of the entire needle trajectory in a single CT image, but the position of the tip of a needle can still be localized adequately. The transoral approach is somewhat awkward when one must leave the room during CT verification, with the needle in the patient's mouth, but has been used with interventional MRI.

Lesions in the pterygopalatine fossa can be approached from above or below the zygomatic arch. Vascular lesions should probably be avoided, because compression is impossible. The authors prefer approaching from above the arch because the downward angle avoids inadvertent entrance into the orbit. Also, skull base lesions have been approached by passing posterior to the carotid artery and styloid process.

Summary

Needle biopsy is an excellent procedure for determining the identity of a mass. Image guidance allows confident sampling and verifies the needle tip position relative to the lesion. The preferred approach and sampling method depend on the site of the lesion and the position of nearby neural and vascular structures.

Further readings

Buckland JR, Manjaly G, Violaris N, et al. Ultrasound-guided cutting-needle biopsy of the parotid gland. J Laryngol Otol 1999;113:988–92.

Curtin HD. Separation of the masticator space from the parapharyngeal space. Radiology 1987;163:195–204.

Duckwiler G, Lufkin RB, Teresi L, et al. Head and neck lesions: MR-guided aspiration biopsy. Radiology 1989;170: 519–22.

Eneroth CM, Hamberger CA. Principles of treatment of different types of parotid tumors. Laryngoscope 1974;84: 1732–40.

Fried MP, Hsu L, Jolesz FA. Interactive magnetic resonance imaging-guided biopsy in the head and neck: initial patient experience. Laryngoscope 1998;108:488–93.

Kesse KW, Manjaly G, Violaris N, et al. Ultrasound-guided biopsy in the evaluation of focal lesions and diffuse swelling of the parotid gland. Br J Oral Maxillofac Surg 2002;40:384–8.

Kletzker GR, Smith PG, Bigelow DC, et al. Management of high parapharyngeal space tumors. Ear Nose Throat J 1991;70:639–47.

Kline TS, Merriam JM, Shapshay SM. Aspiration biopsy cytology of the salivary gland. Am J Clin Pathol 1981;76: 263–9.

Lee MH, Lufkin RB, Borges A, et al. MR-guided procedures using contemporaneous imaging frameless stereotaxis in an open-configuration system. J Comput Assist Tomogr 1998;22:998–1005.

Lewin JS, Petersilge CA, Hatem SF, et al. Interactive MR imaging-guided biopsy and aspiration with a modified clinical C-arm system. AJR Am J Roentgenol 1998;170:1593–601.

Long BW. Image-guided percutaneous needle biopsy: an overview. Radiol Technol 2000;71:335–59.

Mukunyadzi P, Bardales RH, Palmer HE, et al. Tissue effects of salivary gland fine-needle aspiration Does this procedure preclude accurate histologic diagnosis? Am J Clin Pathol 2000;114:741–5.

Nettle WJ, Orell SR. Fine needle aspiration in the diagnosis of salivary gland lesions. Aust N Z J Surg 1989;59:47–51.

Smith OD, Ellis PD, Bearcroft PW, et al. Management of neck lumps–a triage model. Ann R Coll Surg Engl 2000;82: 223–6.

Som PM, Biller HF, Lawson W. Tumors of the parapharyngeal space: preoperative evaluation, diagnosis and surgical approaches. Ann Otol Rhinol Laryngol Suppl 1981;90:3–15.

Som PM, Biller HF, Lawson W, et al. Parapharyngeal space masses: an updated protocol based upon 104 cases. Radiology 1984;153:149–56.

Spearman MP, Curtin HD. CT directed fine needle aspiration of skull base parapharyngeal/infratemporal fossa masses. Skull Base Surgery 1995;5:199–205.

van den Brekel MW, Reitsma LC, Quak JJ, et al. Sonographically guided aspiration cytology of neck nodes for selection of treatment and follow-up in patients with N0 head and neck cancer. AJNR Am J Neuroradiol 1999;20:1727–31.

van den Brekel MW, Castelijns JA, Stel HV, et al. Occult metastatic neck disease: detection with US and US-guided fine-needle aspiration cytology. Radiology 1991;180:457–61.

van den Brekel MW, Castelijns JA, Stel HV, et al. Modern imaging techniques and ultrasound-guided aspiration cytology for the assessment of neck node metastases: a prospective comparative study. Eur Arch Otorhinolaryngol 1993;250:11–7.

Wang SJ, Sercarz JA, Lufkin RB, et al. MRI-guided needle localization in the head and neck using contemporaneous imaging in an open configuration system. Head Neck 2000;22:355–9.

Yamaguchi KT, Strong MS, Shapshay SM, et al. Seeding of parotid carcinoma along Vim-Silverman needle tract. J Otolaryngol 1979;8:49–52.

Yousem DM, Sack MJ, Scanlan KA. Biopsy of parapharyngeal space lesions. Radiology 1994;193:619–22.

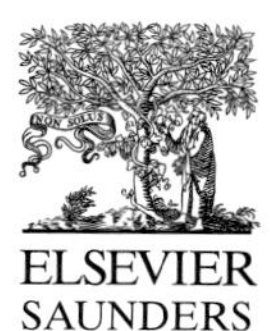

ELSEVIER
SAUNDERS

Atlas Oral Maxillofacial Surg Clin N Am 13 (2005) 63–67

Atlas of the Oral and Maxillofacial Surgery Clinics

Ultrasound Evaluation of Bone Healing in Distraction Osteogenesis of the Mandible

Mary Jane O'Neill, MD

Division of Abdominal Imaging and Interventional Radiology, Massachusetts General Hospital, 55 Fruit Street, White Building, Room 270, Boston, MA 02114, USA

Determining the integrity of the regenerate in the distraction wound is a key factor in the clinical management of patients who undergo mandibular lengthening procedures. The distracters cannot be removed until stiff regenerate bone extends across the distraction gap. The rate of bony healing is difficult to predict and differs from patient to patient; however, because of the lack of adequate imaging assessment of the bone fill within the distraction gap, most surgeons generally use empiric fixation periods before distractor removal. Until recently, no reliable means of estimating the integrity of early bone formation within the mandibular distraction gap has been widely available. The two most common radiographic tests for bony evaluation—plain film and CT—are problematic in this patient population. The immature new bone matrix is difficult to detect reliably on plain radiographs. Although CT attenuation values have been shown to correlate closely with regenerate stability in long bones, artifacts from the distraction devices and dental implants significantly impair CT diagnosis of mandibular wound healing. CT also imparts a relatively high radiation dose to a younger and more radiation-sensitive patient population.

Ultrasound and bone healing

Traditionally, ultrasound has not played a large role in orthopedic diagnosis, but this is rapidly changing with the introduction of new high-resolution linear scanning probes. This new imaging equipment has improved dramatically the ability of ultrasound to evaluate the musculoskeletal system. Although ultrasound assessment of normal mature bone is limited by the inability of the ultrasound beam to penetrate the outer cortex, newly formed bone, which is not completely remodeled and calcified, is well evaluated with high-resolution linear ultrasound [1]. Ultrasound also is a real-time examination, one that can be adapted to the anatomy being examined. This feature allows interrogation of the mandibular distraction gap without interference from the distractors themselves.

Several recent studies have validated the use of ultrasound to assess regenerate integrity by correlating the ultrasound findings with biomechanical tests in animal models [2,3]. These factors allow ultrasound to provide a reliable assessment of the extent of bony healing across the mandibular distraction gap, and the diagnostic findings can be used to time surgical intervention in these patients [4].

E-mail address: moneill@partners.org

1061-3315/05/$ - see front matter
doi:10.1016/j.cxom.2004.12.001

oralmaxsurgeryatlas.theclinics.com

Equipment

Liner high-resolution ultrasound probes of 12 to 15 MHz are required for this examination. Sector probes traditionally used for abdominal and pelvic imaging are inappropriate for this examination because of lower resolution and artifacts related to near field distortion.

Examination technique

The distraction wound is assessed in one primary plane: the plane perpendicular to the osteotomy (Fig. 1). This plane allows identification of the edges of the osteotomy and detailed evaluation of the tissue within the distraction wound. The sonographic evaluation of the wound involves obtaining sequential slices in this plane from the superior to inferior margin of the distraction gap. This plane is established by first identifying the distractors, which are metallic and echogenic and are easily identified in the superficial soft tissues. By elongating the metal distractor, the attachment sites on the proximal and distal bone can be determined. The attachment site of the distractors is usually in close proximity to the edge of the distraction gap, and the plane of the distractor approximates the plane perpendicular to the osteotomy.

Once this plane is established, the probe is moved along the skin on each side of the distractor while maintaining the same imaging plane. This procedure allows visualization of the osteotomy proximal and distal edges and the distraction gap in between. The bone within the gap is evaluated superior and inferior to the distractor, with particular attention paid to the appearance of the proximal and distal bony margin and the integrity of the bone formed within the distraction gap (Fig. 2).

If specific abnormalities are identified or incomplete bone fill-in is suspected, more detailed view of the abnormality can be obtained by interrogating the region in a second plane parallel to the osteotomy plane, but this is generally not required.

Diagnosis of treatment stages

Early in the neutral fixation period after distraction, the wound appears as demonstrated in Fig. 2. Note the well-visualized edges of the distraction gap and the lack of any echogenic material in the wound. The complete through-transmission is sometimes referred to as beam penetration. As healing progresses, islands of echogenic material gradually appear within the

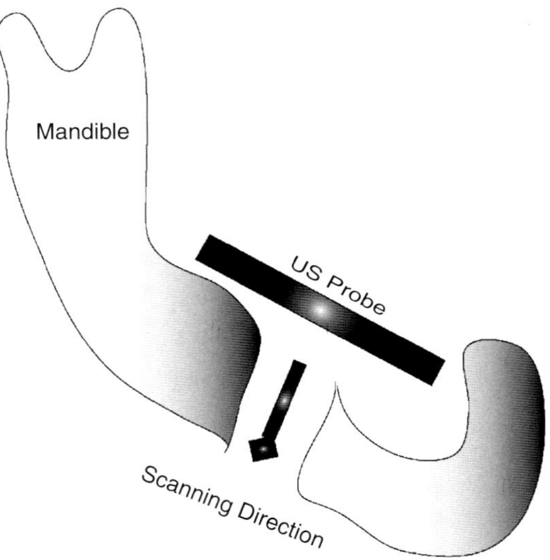

Fig. 1. Schematic representation of probe position in plane perpendicular to the osteotomy. The probe position relative to the distraction wound and the scanning direction is indicated.

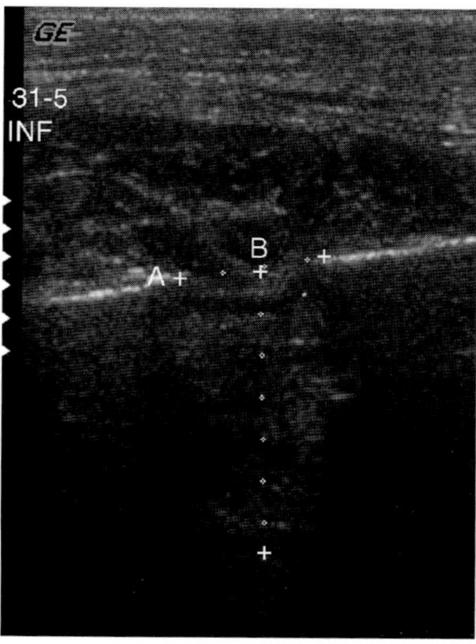

Fig. 2. Longitudinal view perpendicular to the mandibular distraction gap in day 3 of neutral fixation. The cursors labeled A indicate the length of the wound, and the cursors labeled B demonstrate the through-transmission within the wound. No echogenic material in the wound is identified, which indicates lack of new bone formation.

gap (Fig. 3). The echogenic material represents the new bone matrix and is not visualized early in the neutral fixation period of bone distraction. Where the bony islands appear, the ultrasound beam is attenuated and does not penetrate past the echogenic interface of the bone island.

Eventually the islands of bone coalesce and form a complete layer of bridging bone (Fig. 4). The gap edges are less definite at this stage, although a bony depression where the new bone meets the edge of the gap is usually identified, despite the presence of intact bridging bone within the wound. The stage correlates with regenerate stability and signifies the time in which it is safe to remove the distractors [3,4]. As bone healing and remodeling continue, this depression gradually disappears and the wound is indistinguishable from normal cortical bone (Fig. 5).

Patient management

Patients typically undergo imaging after a neutral fixation period that is roughly twice the period of active distraction. At this point most of the wounds demonstrate complete bridging

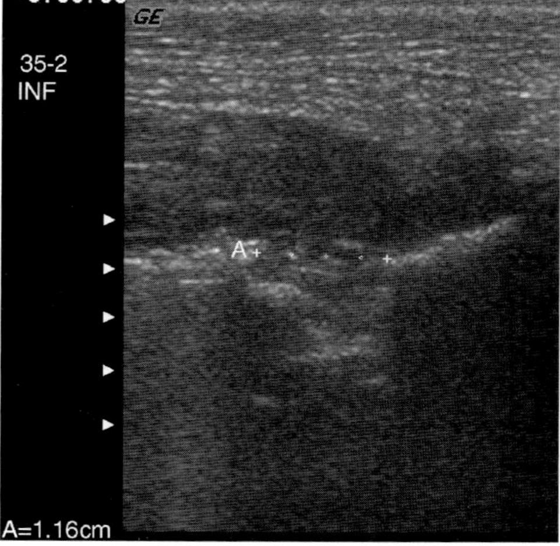

Fig. 3. Longitudinal view perpendicular to the mandibular distraction gap on day 14 of neutral fixation. The cursors labeled A indicate the length of the wound. Note the presence of discontinuous echogenic material in the wound, which indicates the beginning of new bone formation across the gap. The gap edges are still readily visible at this stage.

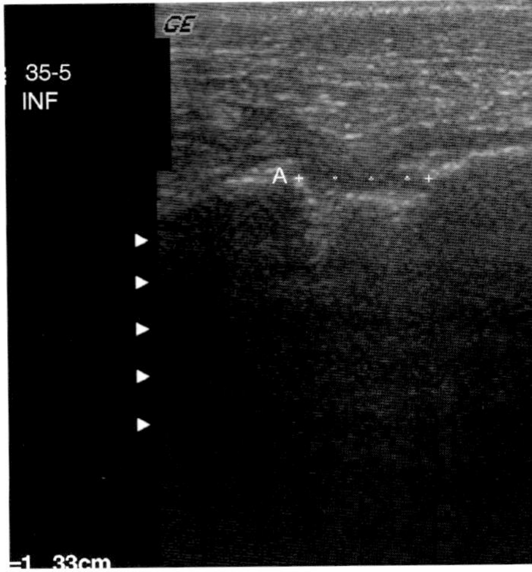

Fig. 4. Longitudinal view perpendicular to the mandibular distraction gap on day 30 of neutral fixation. The cursors labeled A indicate the length of the wound. Note the presence of continuous echogenic material in the wound, which indicates the beginning of new bone formation across the gap. The gap edges are less well defined at this stage. This stage correlates with clinical and biomechanical stability.

bone and distractors can be removed safely. If the wound has not yet healed fully, repeat imaging after a longer neutral period is performed.

Complications

Detection of fluid within the distraction gap and lack of formation of bridging bone despite additional imaging follow-up are atypical findings and usually signify infection and nonunion within the wound.

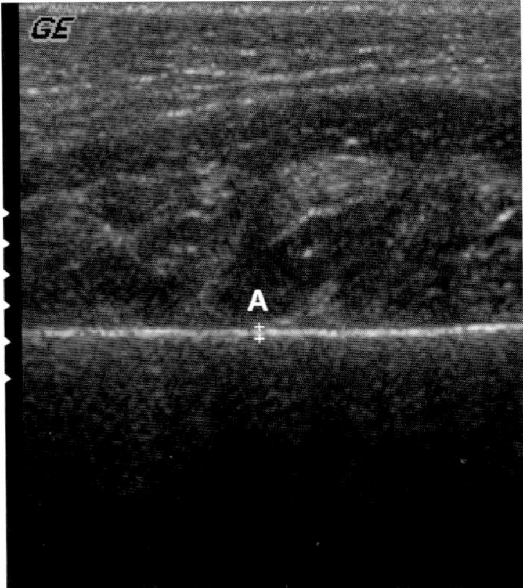

Fig. 5. Longitudinal view perpendicular to the mandibular distraction gap on day 90 after distractor removal. The cursors labeled A indicate the location of mandibular distraction. The new bone is sonographically indistinguishable from the normal adjacent bone.

Summary

Ultrasound is a safe and readily available imaging modality that can predict stability accurately within the wound of patients who undergo mandibular distraction. It is well tolerated by children and adults and does not require sedation for image acquisition. It is relatively free of imaging artifacts produced by the distractors, a problem that affects CT and plain film when used for this assessment. Ultrasound is the optimal imaging modality for assessing mandibular distraction wounds and can be used to help time distractor removal.

References

[1] Derbyshire ND, Simpson AH. A role for ultrasound in limb lengthening. Br J Radiol 1992;775:576–80.

[2] Bail HJ, Kolbeck S, Krummrey G, et al. Ultrasound can predict regenerate stiffness in distraction osteogenesis. Clin Orthop 2002;404:362–7.

[3] Thermuller P, Troulis MJ, O'Neill MJ, et al. Use of ultrasound to assess healing of a mandibular distraction wound. J Oral Maxillofac Surg 2002;60:1038–44.

[4] Troulis MJ, Coppe C, O'Neill MJ, et al. Ultrasound assessment of the distraction osteogenesis wound in patients undergoing mandibular lengthening. J Oral Maxillofac Surg 2003;61:1144–9.

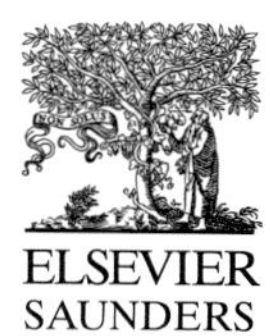

ELSEVIER
SAUNDERS

Atlas Oral Maxillofacial Surg Clin N Am 13 (2005) 69–81

Atlas of the Oral and Maxillofacial Surgery Clinics

Interactive CT Software in Oral and Maxillofacial Surgery

Thomas B. Dodson, DMD, MPH[a,b,*]

[a]*Department of Oral and Maxillofacial Surgery, Massachusetts General Hospital, Boston, MA 02114, USA*
[b]*Department of Oral and Maxillofacial Surgery, Harvard School of Dental Medicine, Boston, MA 02115, USA*

Over the last several years, this author has routinely used desktop computer-based interactive software to view CT studies for the purposes of planning the treatment of endosseous implant cases, managing impacted mandibular third molars (M3s), and as a research tool. This article provides illustrative cases demonstrating how interactive CT imaging facilitates clinical care or research efforts.

Interactive CT imaging software combines the power and detail of CT imaging with the convenience of interacting with the images on a desktop or notebook computer. To a limited degree in some clinical settings, the clinician can work with the radiology technician to interact with CT imaging. The commercially available desktop interactive software permits the clinician to view the radiographic studies in two or three dimensions, make direct measurements, assess bone volumes and density, manipulate the images to simulate implant placement or bone grafting procedures, and simultaneously view the images in the axial, sagittal, and coronal planes.

Although several interactive CT imaging software programs are available, for the purposes of this article, the cases in this article are illustrated using Simplant (Materialise, Glen Burnie, MD). The company made limited licenses available to selected educational institutions to use the software for teaching purposes.

Generally, the process for obtaining the CT images is similar regardless of the system. The patient undergoes a routine CT scan. The CT images are reformatted to be compatible with the interactive software. The images are forwarded to the clinician to view as hard copies or are sent by e-mail or CD media and viewed using the interactive imaging software. Important technical details of acquiring the images vary from system to system and can be obtained by visiting the manufacturer's website or contacting a representative.

Clinical scenario 1: treatment planning for an implant case

Background

Interactive CT software can be a valuable adjunct to planning the treatment of endosseous implant cases. Numerous techniques are available to estimate bony anatomy for implant placement, for example, bone sounding, panoramic or periapical imaging, which includes objects of known size in the image, or transparent implant templates, which are overlayed on the radiographic images. None of these techniques is as powerful or flexible as interactive CT

This work was funded by the Mid-career Investigator's Award in Patient-oriented Research (NIDCR K24 DE000448) and the Department of Oral and Maxillofacial Surgery Education and Research Fund.

* Massachusetts General Hospital, Department of Oral and Maxillofacial Surgery, 55 Fruit Street, Warren 1201, Boston, MA 02114.

E-mail address: tbdodson@partners.org.

1061-3315/05/$ - see front matter
doi:10.1016/j.cxom.2004.11.001

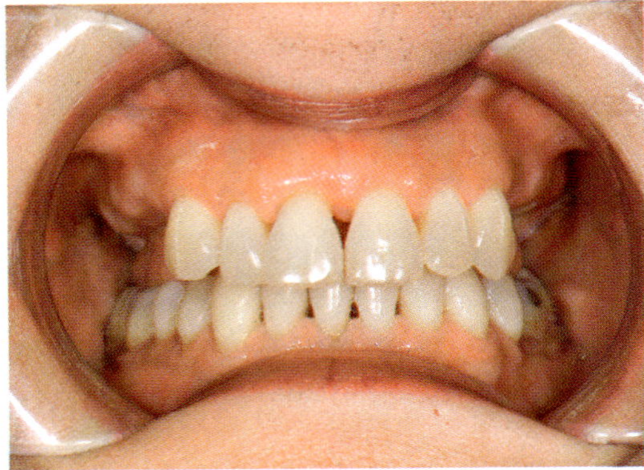

Fig. 1. Intraoral view illustrating the patient's pretreatment dental status. Note the maxillary bilateral posterior edentulous condition.

software for use in diagnosis, treatment planning, and patient education. CT imaging is clearly not needed in all cases to provide excellent patient care and outcomes. In all cases, however, it provides valuable information to increase the chances of good clinical outcomes.

Case presentation 1

The patient is a 52-year-old female who presented for an evaluation for dental implants to facilitate restoration of her posterior maxilla, using implant-based fixed prostheses (Fig. 1).

Treatment planning images

To complete the treatment planning process, the patient was scheduled for a CT scan of her maxilla, with reformatting of the images to facilitate use with the interactive CT viewing software. To facilitate treatment planning, the restorative dentist fabricated a surgical stent with the planned prostheses ideally positioned. A radio-opaque material such as gutta percha was inserted in the desired implant sites. The completed template was worn at the time the CT images were acquired (Fig. 2).

Fig. 3 is a representative view of the reformatted CT images using the interactive CT imaging software. The upper right view shows the level of the axial CT cut. The lower right image shows the corresponding panoramic view and the radio-opaque implant markers from the surgical template. The images on the right side of the screen are the coronal images (cross-sectional views).

Fig. 4 is a representative view of the reformatted CT image being used to develop the treatment plan for an implant in the region of the maxillary right first bicuspid. The software

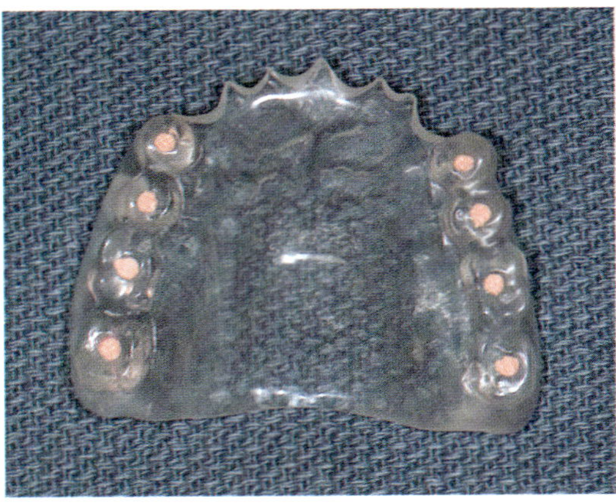

Fig. 2. Proposed surgical template worn at the time of the CT imaging. Note the radio-opaque material, gutta percha in this case, centered in the planned implant sites.

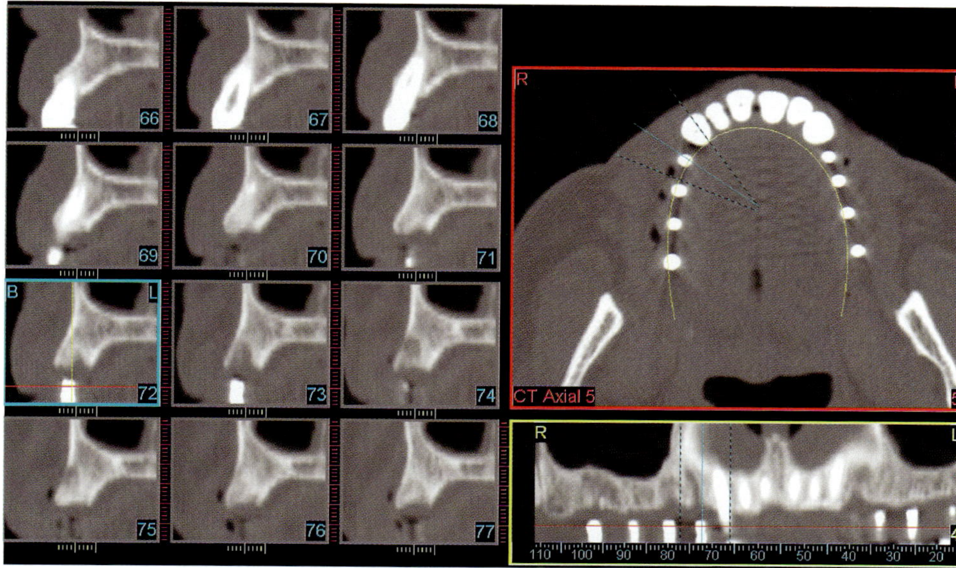

Fig. 3. A typical view available with the interactive CT software. At the upper right is the axial CT scan showing the position of the planned restorations. At the lower right is the corresponding panoramic view showing seven of the eight planned implants. The eighth implant (position of *upper left* second molar) is outside the plane of the reformatted panoramic image (see the *yellow line* in the *upper right* image). The red line in the panoramic view corresponds to the level of the axial CT view in the upper right. At the left are 12 coronal views proceeding from the anterior (*upper left*) to posterior (*lower right*), centered about the restoration for the maxillary right first bicuspid. The blue lines on the axial CT image outline the area detailed in the coronal view. This view permits the clinician to view the case in all three-dimensions simultaneously.

includes a measuring tool to estimate the height and width of available bone. As seen in Fig. 4, the estimated height and width of available bone was 16 and 10 mm, respectively. The implant could be as long as 15 mm and still engage native bone. Fig. 4 illustrates the placement of a 4.00 mm × 15.00 mm implant at the site of the maxillary right first bicuspid. One feature of the software is that it contains an implant library permitting the clinician to select an available implant from a manufacturer and to specify the dimensions (ie, diameter and length) as well.

The software also permits treatment planning for bone grafts. Fig. 5 simulates a bone graft being placed in the right maxillary sinus to permit a longer implant to be placed at site 3 (maxillary right first molar). Fig. 5 illustrates a case after simulating placement of eight implants with a focused view of the upper right quadrant and the bone graft. Volume estimates of grafted needed are also provided.

After careful case treatment planning, how is the plan transferred from the computer to the patient? Companies such as Materialise are able to fabricate surgical stents based on the treatment plan, which permit precise placement of implants in three dimensions. Fig. 6 shows the prefabricated surgical stents on a three-dimensional model developed from the treatment plan. Fig. 7 shows the set of stents, from the pilot holes to the final drill sizes, used to complete the implant osteotomies. Fig. 8 is a panoramic radiograph of the case, obtained immediately after implant placement.

Clinical scenario 2: management of impacted M3s

Background

An uncommon but distressing complication of removing impacted M3s is an inferior alveolar nerve (IAN) or lingual nerve injury. Although there are anatomic guidelines for locating the lingual nerve, there currently are no imaging techniques available to identify lingual nerve position. The IAN, however, can be routinely visualized using standard panoramic radiographs,

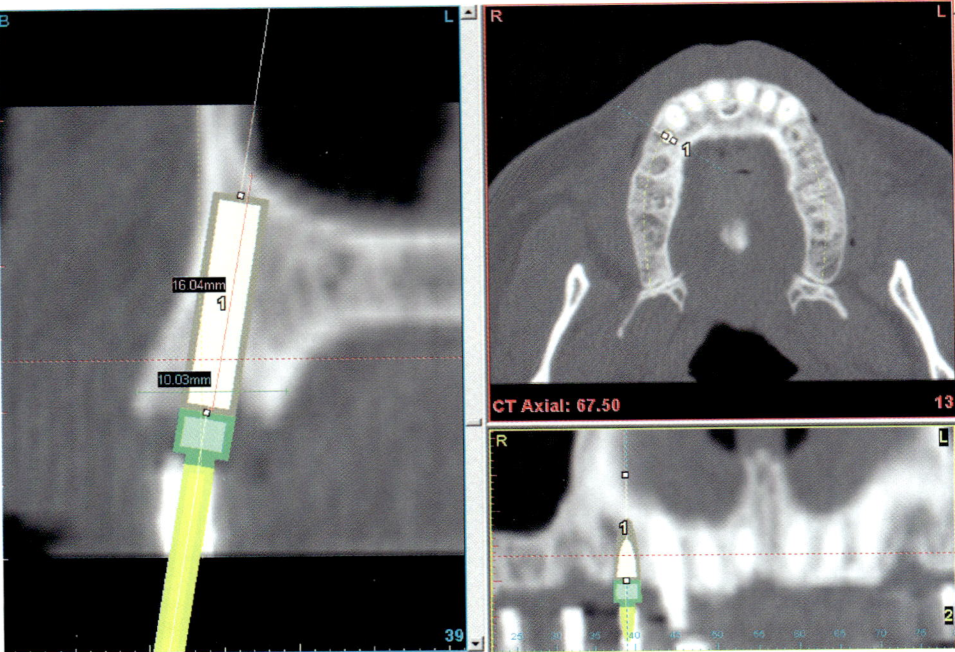

Fig. 4. A typical view after placing the planned implant (1) in the site of the upper right maxillary first bicuspid. A software measuring tool helps to quantify the available bone in terms of height and width. In this case, on the left hand side of the image, the solid red line marks the bone height (16 mm), and the solid green line marks the bone width (10 mm). The placement of a 4.0 × 15-mm implant is simulated.

and there is a set of radiographic findings that are associated with increased risks for IAN injury (Fig. 9). Based on reviews of the literature and the authors research, it seems that in the setting in which there are no visible signs of increased risk on the panoramic radiograph, the risk of IAN injury is small (≤1%) [1–3].

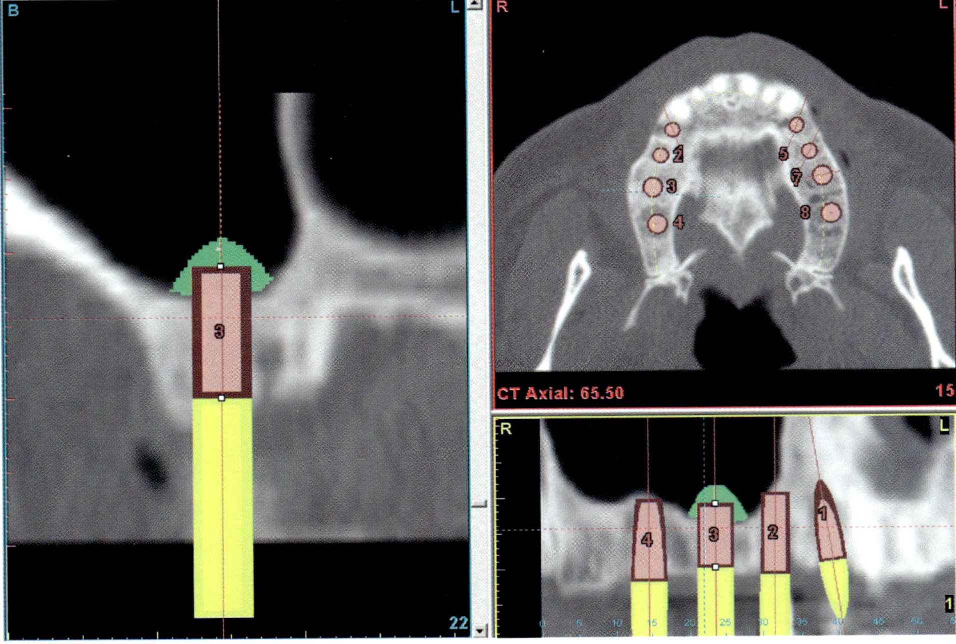

Fig. 5. An overview after all eight implants have been "placed" (*upper right*). The lower right image shows the condition in the upper right quadrant after the implants have been placed and a simulated bone graft (green) has been inserted. The left image is a coronal view of implant 3 and its associated bone graft.

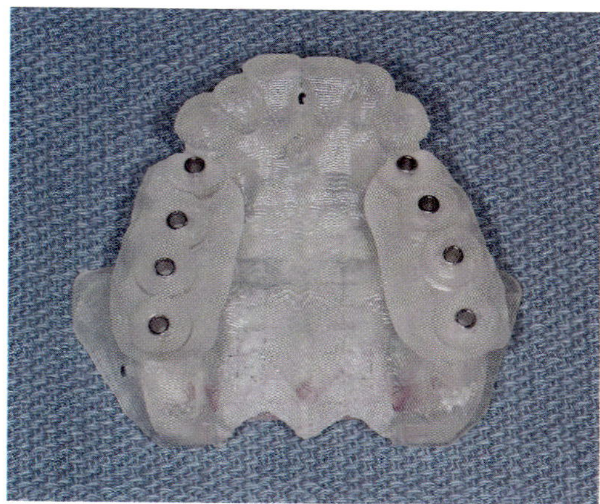

Fig. 6. The bone-supported surgical template in position on a three-dimensional model that was fabricated based on the computerized treatment plan.

The baseline risk of IAN injury, absent any radiographic information, is approximately 1%. In the setting of positive panoramic radiographic findings associated with an increased risk for IAN injury, the risk of IAN injury is still unlikely but increases from a baseline of 1% to 1.4% to 12% [2]. In clinical practice, it is rare to rely on only one fact or finding to make decisions. In the setting of high-risk findings, additional imaging is recommended [2–4]. Suggested alternative imaging modalities include periapical films or tomography. In the author's practice, when concerned about the risk of IAN injury arises, a CT scan is ordered, with the images reformatted so they can be viewed with interactive CT software.

Not all patients benefit from preoperative CT imaging. The decision to routinely scan all patients is a thoughtless, medico-legal exercise resulting in unnecessary radiation exposure and expense, with no evidence that imaging predictably decreases the risk of IAN injury after M3 removal. The more challenging decision is in selecting the patients that may benefit from the incremental radiation exposure and cost of a limited CT scan. In assessing the risk of IAN injury after M3 extraction, the clinician consciously or unconsciously incorporates multiple radiographic findings into the decision-making process, for example, the degree of root development, anatomic position of M3, overall degree of extraction difficulty, and type and number of positive radiographic signs. In the study by Sedaghatfar et al [3], the surgeons' overall clinical impression based on radiographic findings had the highest positive and negative predictive values relative to the radiographic findings alone when trying to predict the risk of IAN nerve exposure at the time of M3 removal.

A parameter this author considers in the case of a high-risk patient (ie, a patient with one or more panoramic radiographic findings suggesting an increased risk for IAN injury) is whether M3 extraction is most likely unavoidable because of symptoms. In this setting, using interactive CT software is valuable for localizing the position of the IAN relative to the M3 to assess the

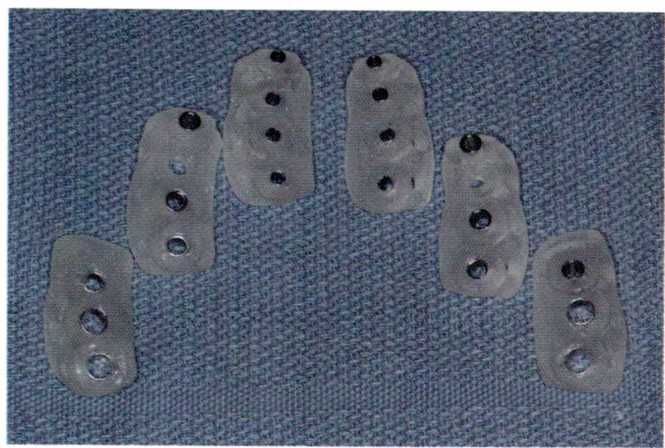

Fig. 7. Set of surgical templates produced to guide the osteotomies from the pilot holes to the final osteotomies.

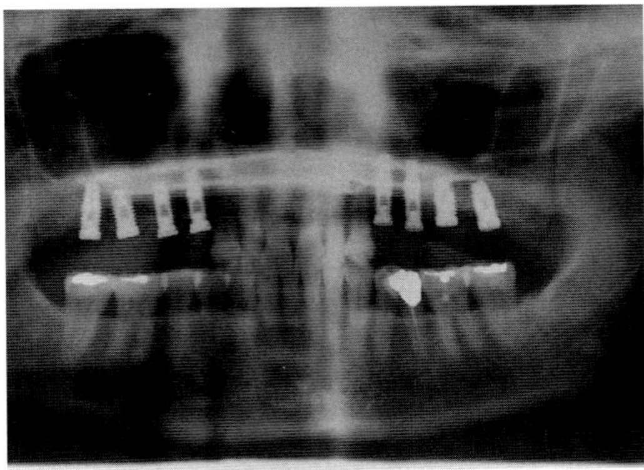

Fig. 8. Panoramic radiograph illustrating the implant positions at the end of the case.

risk for IAN injury. Additionally, knowledge of IAN position provides the operator with the opportunity to plan the operation to minimize the risk for IAN injury. For example, if it is known that the IAN is located to the lingual of the tooth, the operation can proceed quickly, efficiently, and aggressively from the buccal approach, with confidence that there is little risk to the nerve. Alternatively, in a patient with a history, physical examination, and radiographic examination of an asymptomatic impacted M3 who shows panoramic findings of increased IAN injury risk, interactive CT software tools can help to localize the IAN and assess the risk for IAN injury. Given the low risk of IAN injury, the patient may elect to proceed with treatment. The clinician can then execute the operation with full confidence of knowing the IAN location. Given a high risk of IAN injury, the patient may elect to treat the M3 with annual monitoring.

Case presentation 2

The patient was a 25-year-old female who had two impacted mandibular M3s that were asymptomatic, by history. The physical examination was remarkable for the absence of any

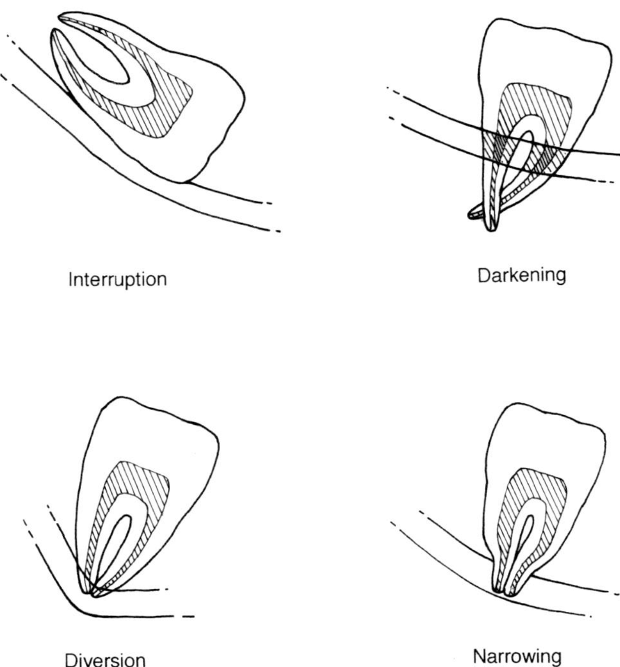

Fig. 9. Examples of panoramic radiographic findings associated with an increased risk for IAN injury after M3 removal. (*Upper left*) Interruption or loss of the white cortical line corresponding to the IAN canal. (*Upper right*) Darkening of the M3 root as the IAN canal crosses the root. (*Lower left*) Diversion of the IAN canal as it passes the M3 root. (*Lower right*) Narrowing of the M3 root apex as the IAN canal crosses the root.

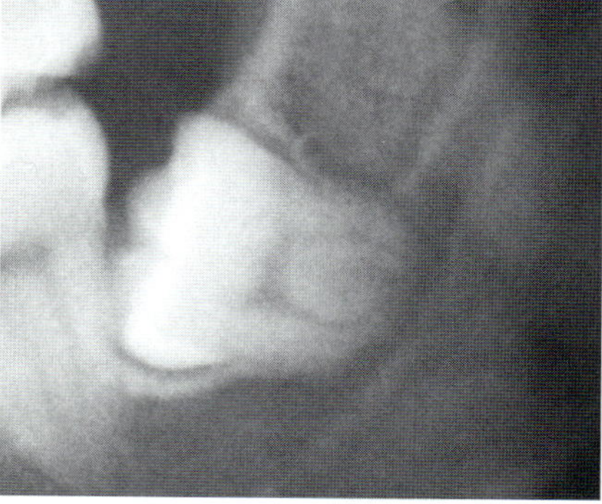

Fig. 10. Panoramic radiograph focused on the mandibular left M3. Superimposition of the M3 over the IAN canal, loss of the superior cortical margin of the IAN canal, and narrowing of the canal are shown.

pathology. The mandibular M3s were completely covered with mucosa and could not be probed with a periodontal probe, and probing depths on the distal of the mandibular second molar were 2 to 3 mm. Panoramic radiographic imaging was negative for pathology. Findings on panoramic imaging, however, showed a loss of the superior cortical margin of the IAN canal adjacent to the mandibular left M3, that is, a loss of the white line and narrowing of the IAN canal as it crossed the apices of the M3 roots (Fig. 10).

In summary, the patient had impacted mandibular M3s that were by history, physical, and radiographic examination, asymptomatic. There were radiographic findings, however, suggesting that the patient was at increased risk for IAN injury. The patient was offered the choice of M3 extraction or continued follow-up on an annual basis to monitor the M3s, with extraction planned if and when the M3s became symptomatic. The patient was interested in extraction but was concerned about the risk for IAN injury and elected to undergo further imaging studies, that is, CT, with reformatting for interactive CT viewing.

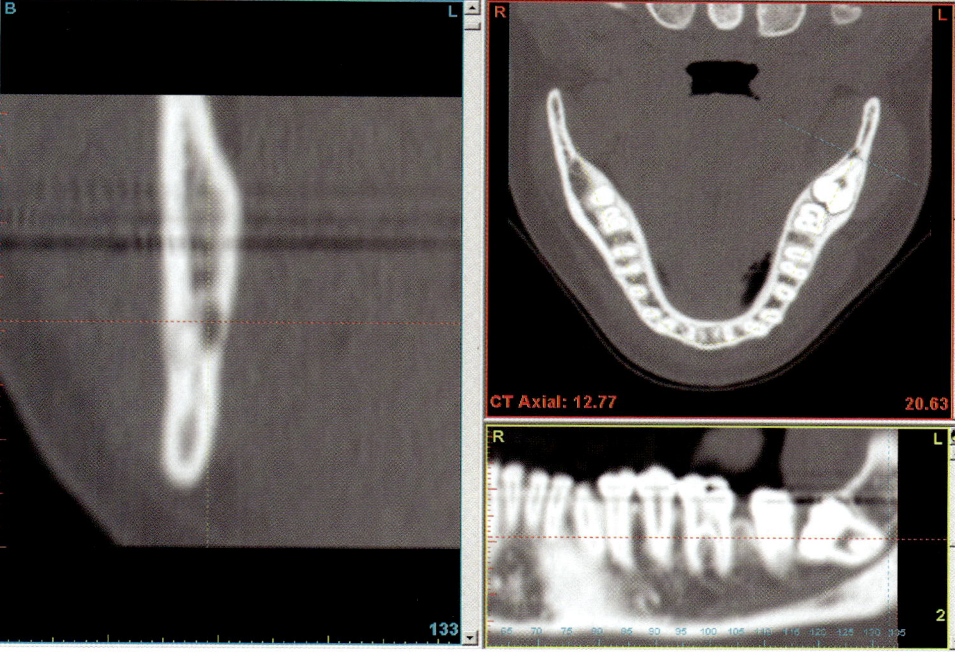

Fig. 11. The crosshairs of a proximal reformatted CT image are centered over the middle of the IAN canal at the M3 apex. The IAN canal is clearly separate from the M3 and lingual to the apex (see Fig. 12).

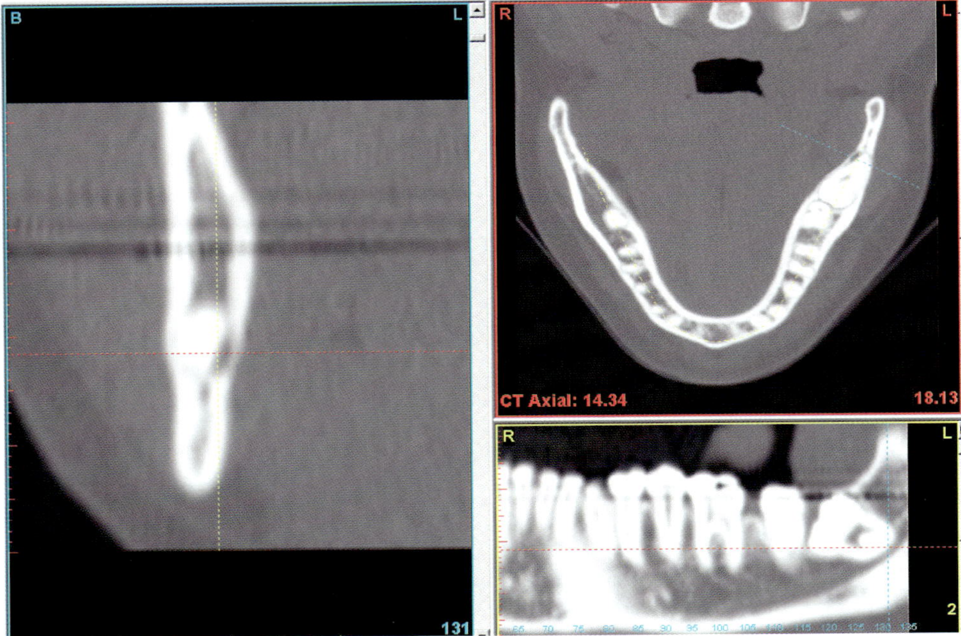

Fig. 12. The IAN canal appears compressed, separate from the M3, and positioned medially to the M3 (see Fig. 13).

Reformatted CT images

Figs. 11–13 illustrate the relationship of the IAN canal as it passes from proximal to distal in the region of the left M3. Fig. 11 clearly shows the IAN canal adjacent and lingual to the M3 apex. Figs. 12 and 13 demonstrate the IAN canal passing adjacent and lingual to the M3 before diving inferiorly to the M3.

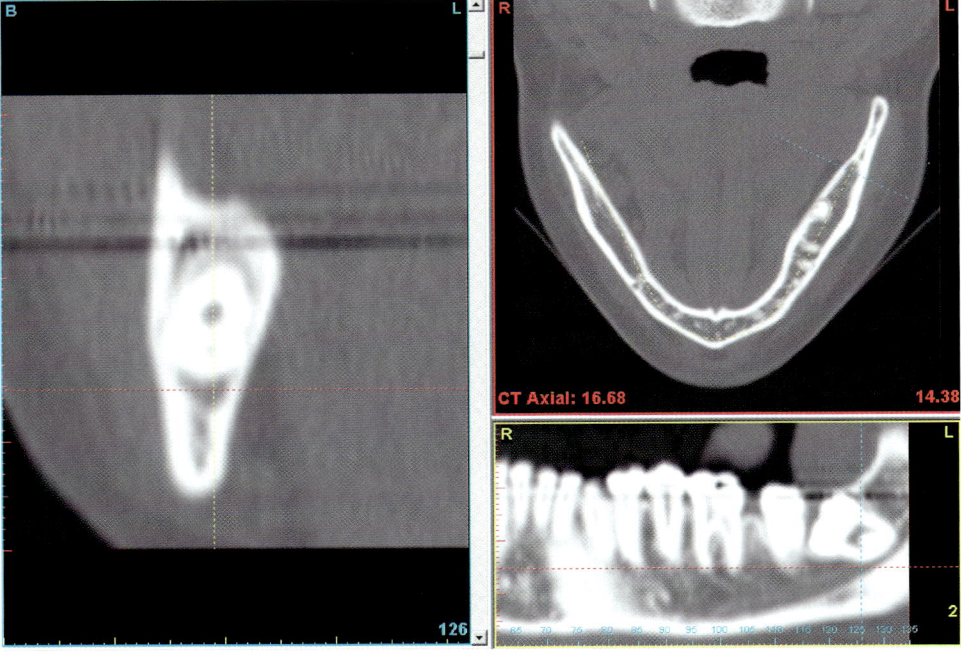

Fig. 13. The IAN canal appears inferiorly to the M3 and has begun to move laterally.

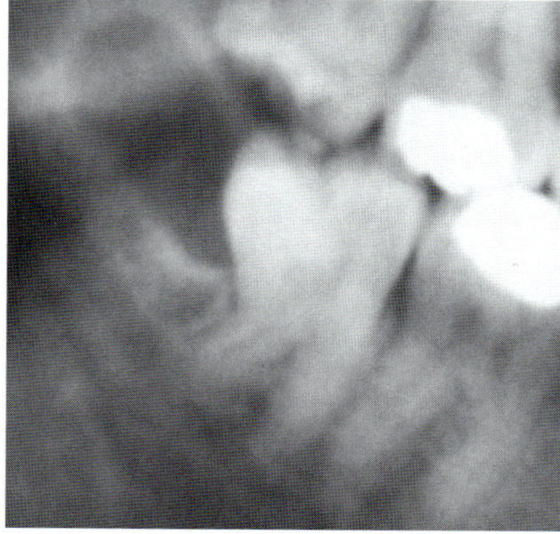

Fig. 14. Mandibular right M3. Note evidence of a radiolucent lesion proximal to the tooth, loss of the superior border of the IAN canal, and darkening of the mesial root.

Clinical decision summary and outcome

After reviewing the reformatted CT images, given M3 removal, the risk for a temporary IAN injury was estimated to be higher than average, given the proximity of the IAN to the M3 apex. Because the position of the IAN relative to the M3 was known, however, the tooth could be approached safely from the buccal, keeping the M3 between the drill and the IAN, and the M3 could be removed with little risk of a permanent IAN injury. Therefore, it was recommended that the M3 be removed. After M3 removal, the IAN was visualized at the apical, lingual position of the extraction site, consistent with the preoperative imaging, and was noted to be intact. The patient recovered without incident.

Case presentation 3

The patient was a 32-year-old female who was self-referred for the evaluation of her M3s. She had a history of intermittent pain and discomfort but was currently asymptomatic. On physical

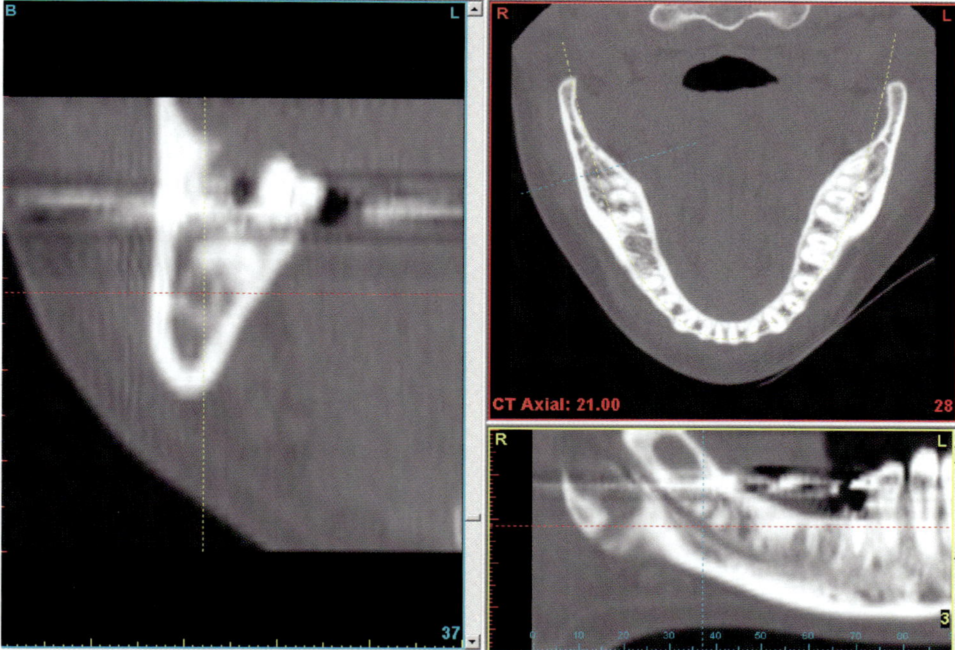

Fig. 15. Reformatted CT image with the crosshairs centered over the IAN canal. The canal appears to be inferior and lateral to the tooth.

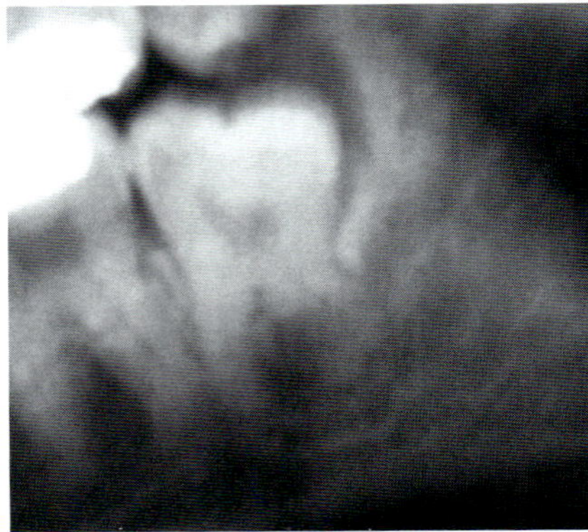

Fig. 16. Mandibular left M3. Note superimposition of the IAN canal and the M3 roots, loss of the cortical margins of the IAN canal, and darkening of the root.

examination, both mandibular M3s were partially erupted, associated with inflamed soft tissue, and had purulent drainage. Panoramic radiographic imaging revealed a 1.5-cm cystic lesion on the distal of the mandibular right M3 (Figs. 14, 15). Additionally, both M3s had radiographic findings associated with an increased risk for IAN injury (see Fig. 14) (Fig. 16). The mandibular right M3 showed a loss of the superior cortical margin (white line), the IAN canal, and darkening of the mesial root (see Fig. 14). The mandibular left M3 showed a superimposition of the IAN canal and M3, loss of the superior margin of the IAN canal, and darkening of the midroot of M3 (see Fig. 16). Because the patient most likely would need operative intervention to manage her M3s, the author recommended she undergo preoperative CT imaging reformatted for interactive viewing.

Reformatted CT images

After reviewing the reformatted images of the right M3 (Fig. 15), the risk of IAN injury was believed to be low. The IAN canal passed inferiorly and buccal to the apices of the M3. In

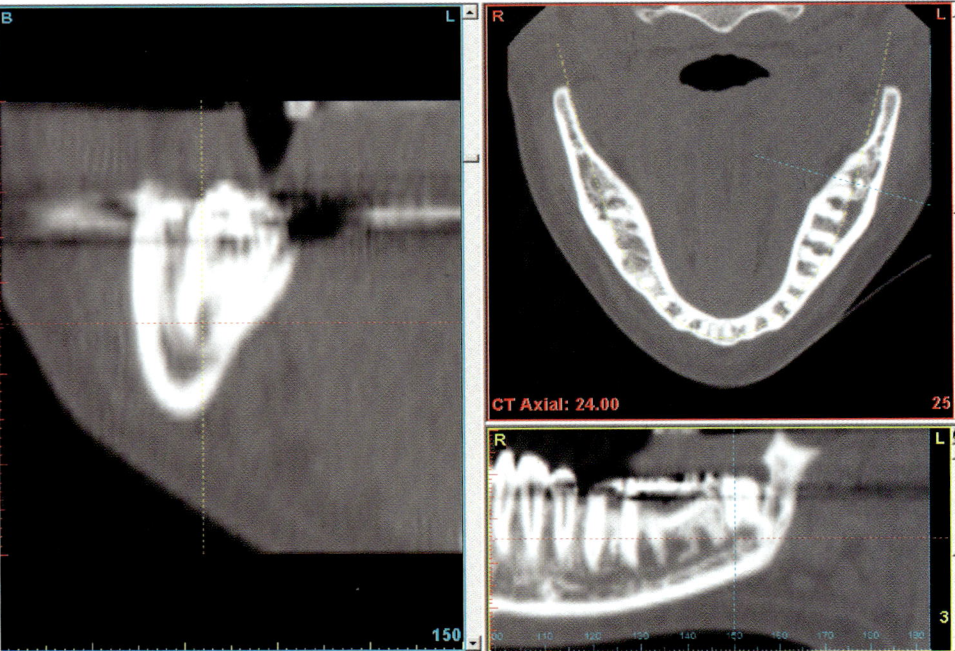

Fig. 17. Reformatted CT image with the crosshairs centered on the IAN canal at the position of the mesial root of the mandibular left M3.

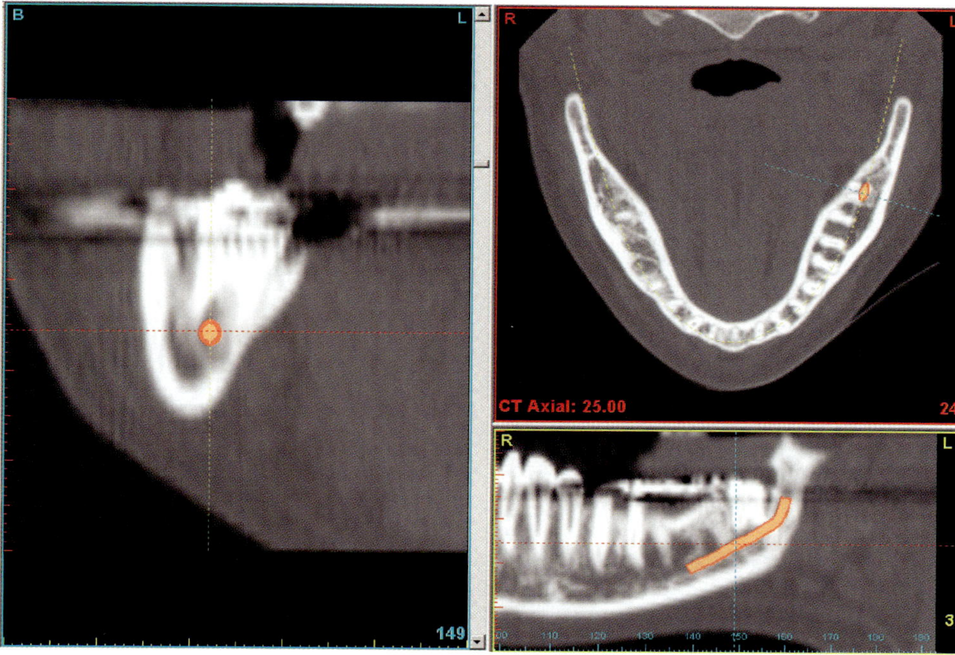

Fig. 18. Reformatted CT image demonstrates the use of a software tool to trace the path of the IAN canal as it passes through the mandible. The IAN canal can be seen passing laterally to the M3 distal root and between the bifurcation or substance of the mesial M3 root.

contrast, the risk of IAN injury was estimated to be high on the left M3. The IAN canal appears to be passing through the substance of the mesial root or a bifurcation of the mesial root (Fig. 17). Using an available software tool, it was possible to trace the IAN canal (Fig. 18).

Clinical decision and outcomes

Given the evidence of a radiolucent lesion associated with the mandibular right M3 and the low risk of IAN injury associated with M3 removal and excision of the lesion, it was an easy decision to recommend extraction of the right M3.

Management of the mandibular left M3, however, presented a more difficult decision. On the one hand, pathology was present (ie, caries and chronic pericoronitis with acute exacerbations). Given the CT findings, however, the risk for a serious IAN injury after M3 extraction appeared high and possibly inevitable.

On the day of the procedure, the radiographic findings and treatment options were reviewed with the patient. She perceived the right M3 as being a serious issue and consented to its removal. She deferred extraction of the left M3 and elected restorative and periodontal care and annual evaluations of the situation. The mandibular M3 and associated soft tissue lesion, an inflamed dentigerous cyst, were removed without complication. The postoperative course was unremarkable.

The prognosis of the left M3 is guarded at best, and the decision to retain it probably will only result in deferring the final treatment decision. At some point in the future, the M3 in this case will need operative intervention. A decision will need to be made whether to extract the M3 or to perform a coronectomy [5–7].

Research scenario: systematic assessment of the IAN position

Background

There are several anatomic studies [8,9,10] of cadaveric specimens that document intrabony IAN anatomy and position [8,9]. In virtually all of these studies, however, there were no

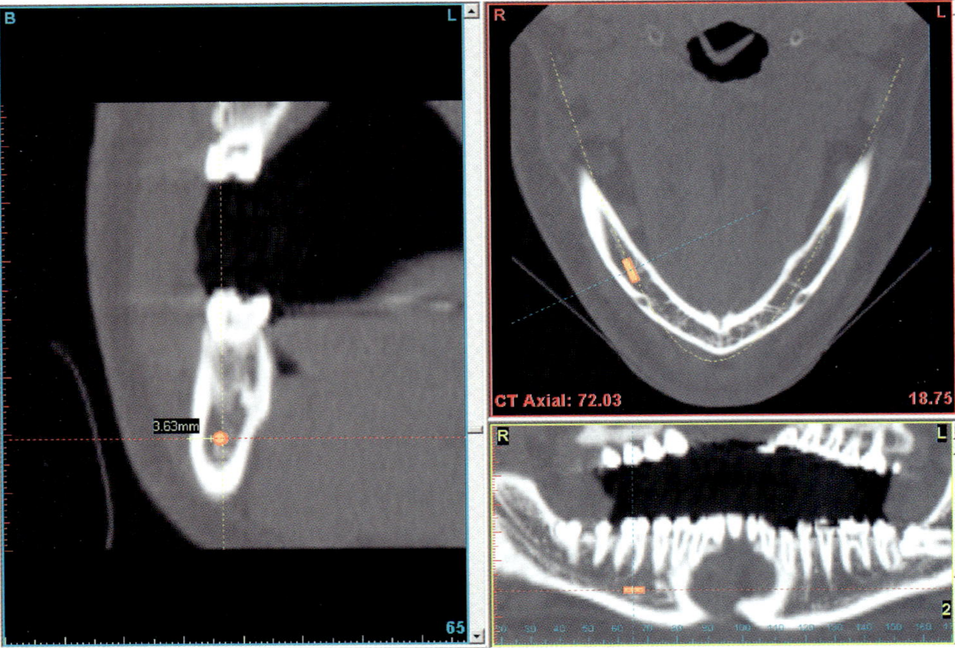

Fig. 19. Reformatted CT image showing the use of the software for research purposes. The IAN has been traced, and at the position of the bifurcation of the mandibular first molar, the distance between the canal and lateral cortical border of the mandible can be measured using an available software tool.

demographic data available to assess the influence of variables such as age, sex, or ethnicity on IAN position. In an attempt to redress this deficiency in the literature, the present author applied interactive CT software technology to describe the position of the IAN in a clinically relevant location, that is, the region of the mandibular first molar, a location where the vertical limb of a sagittal split osteotomy or a monocortical bone screw may be placed, and to identify patient-specific factors that were associated with IAN position [10].

The study was designed as a retrospective study and used a convenience sample of subjects who had undergone mandibular axial CT imaging that was reformatted for viewing with the Simplant Planner. The predictor variables were patient-specific factors, including age, gender, and race. The outcome variable was the distance between the outer buccal cortical margin and the outer cortical buccal margin of the mandible. The distance was estimated using the measuring tool available with Simplant Planner (Fig. 19).

The sample consisted of 50 subjects. On average, the buccal aspect of the mandible was located 4.9 mm (range, 1.3–7.8 mm) from the buccal margin of the canal. For purposes of comparison, the maximum diameter of the fluted Lindemann bur is 2.0 mm and tapers to 1.5 mm. On average, as age increased, the distance decreased ($P = 0.04$) from the IAN canal to the buccal cortex. The position of the nerve also decreased in distance from the buccal cortex in whites when compared with nonwhites ($P = 0.04$).

Summary

This article illustrates the role of interactive CT software to facilitate the management of patients who require implant placement or M3 extraction and for research. Not all patients require CT imaging. There is a subset of patients, however, who may benefit from incremental imaging. In the author's practice, using interactive CT imaging is considered for implant patients who require bone grafts, placement of multiple adjacent implants, or if the IAN may be at risk for injury. For M3 patients who have multiple risk factors for IAN injury based on a review of the panoramic radiograph will be considered for CT imaging. Additionally, there is a small subset of patients who request preoperative CT imaging. Finally, there is a role for interactive CT image for research purposes in which direct measurements on living subjects are desirable.

References

[1] Rood JP, Nooraldeen Shehab BAA. The radiological prediction of inferior alveolar nerve injury during third molar surgery. Br J Oral Maxillofac Surg 1990;28:20–5.
[2] Blaeser BF, August MA, Donoff RB, et al. Panoramic radiographic risk factors for inferior alveolar nerve injury after third molar extraction. J Oral Maxillofac Surg 2003;61(4):417–21.
[3] Sedaghatfar M, August M, Dodson TB. Panoramic radiographic findings and the risk for inferior alveolar nerve injury following third molar extraction. J Oral Maxillofac Surg 2002;60(Suppl 1):S100.
[4] Monaco G, Montevecchi M, Bonetti G, et al. Reliability of panoramic radiography in evaluating the topographic relationship between the mandibular canal and impacted third molars. J Am Dent Assoc 2004;135:312–8.
[5] Pogrel MA, Lee JS, Muff DF. Coronectomy in lower third molar surgery. J Oral Maxillofac Surg 2003;61(Suppl 1): S25.
[6] Knutsson K, Lysell I, Rohlin M. Postoperative status after partial removal of the mandibular third molar. Swed Dent J 1989;13:15–22.
[7] Freedman GL. Intentional partial odontectomy. J Oral Maxillfac Surg 1997;55:524–6.
[8] Yang J, Cavalcanti MG, Ruprecht A, et al. 2-D and 3-D reconstructions of spiral computed tomography in localization of the inferior alveolar canal for dental implants. Oral Surg Oral Med Oral Pathol 1999;87:369–74.
[9] da Fontoura RA, Vasconcellos HA, Campos AE. Morphologic basis for the intraoral vertical ramus osteotomy: anatomic and radiographic localization of the mandibular foramen. J Oral Maxillofac Surg 2002;60:660–5.
[10] Levine MH, Goddard AL, Dodson TB. Inferior alveolar nerve canal position. A clinical and radiographic study. J Oral Maxillofac Surg 2003;61(Suppl 1):S72.

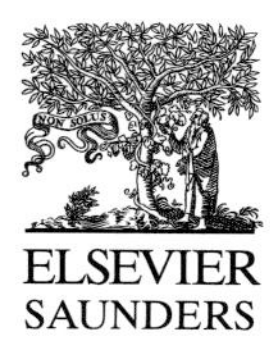
ELSEVIER
SAUNDERS

Atlas Oral Maxillofacial Surg Clin N Am 13 (2005) 83–89

Atlas of the Oral and Maxillofacial Surgery Clinics

Custom-Made Total Temporomandibular Joint Prostheses

David A. Keith, BDS, FDSRCS, DMD

Department of Oral and Maxillofacial Surgery, Massachusetts General Hospital, Harvard School of Dental Medicine, 55 Fruit Street, Warren 1201, Boston, MA 02114, USA

Postoperative management

Long-term prognosis

In the multiply operated patient and patients with severe anatomic problems that involve the temporomandibular joint, total temporomandibular joint reconstruction with a prosthesis may be necessary. The various systems available currently are discussed in a previous issue of the *Oral and Maxillofacial Surgery Clinics of North America*. This article discusses the general principles involved in total temporomandibular joint replacement. The choice of which system to use is left to the preference of the individual oral and maxillofacial surgeon.

Indications

Severe mandibular hypomobility is a result of bony ankylosis or is secondary to adhesions across the joint and the joint space. Ankylosis is the end stage of a process initiated by trauma, inflammation, infection, radiation, or previous surgery. Progressive bony and soft-tissue changes gradually limit the range of motion until eventually the jaw becomes completely immobile. This process may or may not be accompanied by pain. The cause depends on several factors. Historically and currently in areas with limited health care resources, infection is a major cause of ankylosis. Trauma is a frequent etiologic factor, and currently, the multiply operated patient is the leading candidate for total joint replacement. Severe destructive changes are seen in cases of rheumatoid arthritis and ankylosing spondylitis and in idiopathic condylysis and foreign body giant cell reaction to implant materials. Loss of tissue may occur in ablative surgery or after trauma.

Patient assessment

Medical

A patient's medical history should be reviewed in detail. Allergy to the components of the prosthesis, active infection in the surgical site, and medical conditions are absolute contra-indications.

E-mail address: dkeith@partners.org

doi:10.1016/j.cxom.2004.12.003

Psychological

Many patients with temporomandibular disorders and especially patients who have undergone multiple surgeries suffer chronic pain and may have comorbid depression or anxiety. The outcomes must be discussed with patients and include expectations about continuing pain and range of motion. The surgeon may need to refer a patient to a behavioral health specialist and a pain management specialist to assess and support the patient through the perioperative period.

Imaging studies

Surgeons are aided by three-dimensional imaging. Reconstructed three-dimensional CT scans with 1-mm cuts are helpful in delineating the extent of bony ankylosis and bone overgrowth as they invade the base of the skull, glenoid fossa, and zygomatic arch. Frequently, excess bone is present on the medial aspect of the joint or impinges on the external auditory meatus. In destructive conditions, perforations may be present through the glenoid fossa into the middle cranial fossa. The anatomy of the mandibular ramus also must be evaluated, because it receives the condylar prosthesis. Stereolithographic models are invaluable in guiding a surgeon in the removal of the bony mass and planning the design of the custom-made prosthesis. These images are also used to assess the shape and size of the coronoid process, which in long-standing cases of mandibular hypomobility may become elongated and impinge on the zygomatic area and prevent full mobilization of the mandible.

Surgery

The key principle is to mobilize completely the mandible at the time of surgery. Inevitably and despite vigorous physical therapy, the long-term range of motion achieved is less than that obtained in the operating room. The temporomandibular joint is approached by way of standard preauricular and submandibular incisions. In cases of ankylosis, hemi-coronal, or in bilateral cases, a coronal flap provides better access and visualization of the surgical site, including the medial aspect of the joint and the coronoid process.

One-stage surgery

In cases in which the anatomy of the glenoid fossa and mandibular ramus has not been altered significantly by disease or prior surgery, off-the-shelf total joints of varying shapes and sizes can be fitted. In most cases of ankylosis, the anatomy has been so distorted that custom-designed prostheses are necessary. This article concentrates on this situation.

Initial assessment

A patient with severe mandibular hypomobility is assessed by history, physical examination, including range of motion measurements, and plain films (Fig. 1). If the initial evaluation suggests a diagnosis of temporomandibular joint ankylosis, a CT scan is ordered (Fig. 2). The scan assesses (1) condition of the temporomandibular joints, (2) the shape and size of the coronoid processes, (3) the anatomy of the zygomatic arches, (4) the condition of the base of the skull, (5) the length of the styloid process and its possible fusion to the mandible, (6) the condition of the native mandibular ramus and body, and (7) the relationship of the maxilla and mandible.

MRI studies also may be necessary to assess the condition of the contralateral temporomandibular joint, which, in the case of trauma, may demonstrate fibrous ankylosis without significant osseous change. To achieve full mobilization, this condition must be addressed at the same time that the mandible is mobilized.

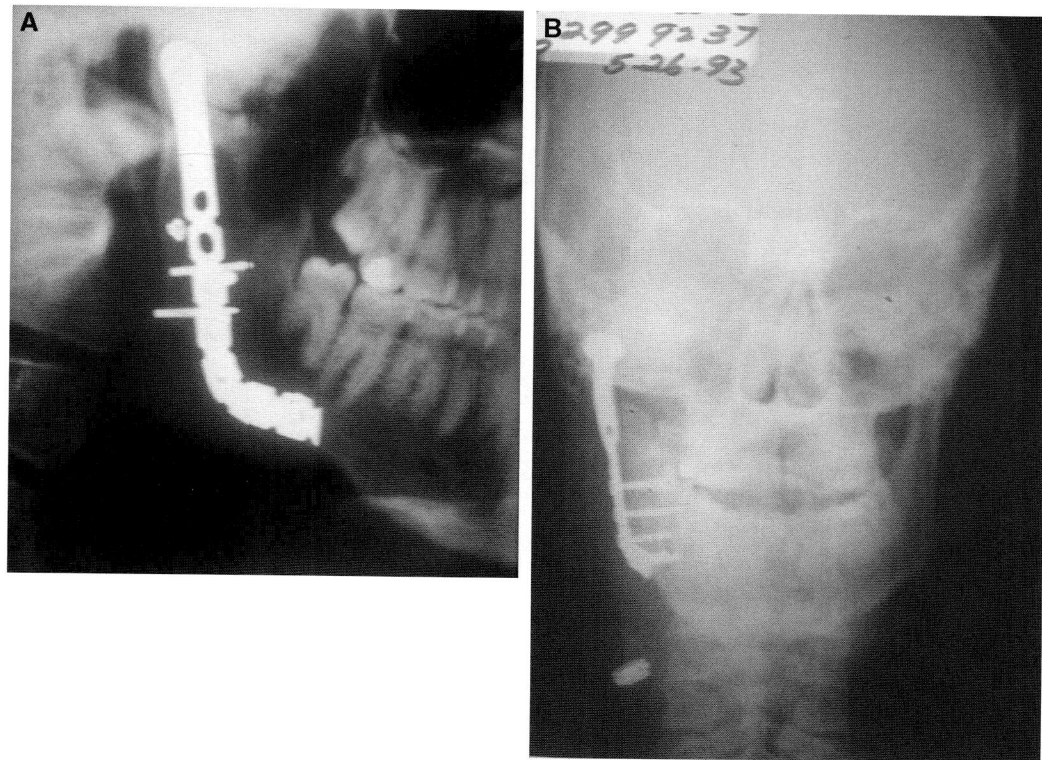

Fig. 1. Panoramic (*A*) and anterior-posterior (*B*) cephalogram of a patient who had a right condylar fracture at age 8 years. He subsequently developed bony ankylosis, and a costochondral graft was placed. The bony ankylosis recurred. The ankylotic mass was excised, and a condylar reconstruction plate was placed. The ankylosis recurred.

Treatment sequencing

Mobilization of the mandible entails (1) excision of the ankylotic mass from the base of the skull down to the level of mandibular lingula (Fig. 3), (2) removal of the coronoid process, (3) excision of the stylohyoid ligament, and (4) stripping of scarred soft tissue and muscle. In bilateral cases, these procedures must be performed on both sides. In unilateral cases, the contralateral coronoid process may need to be removed.

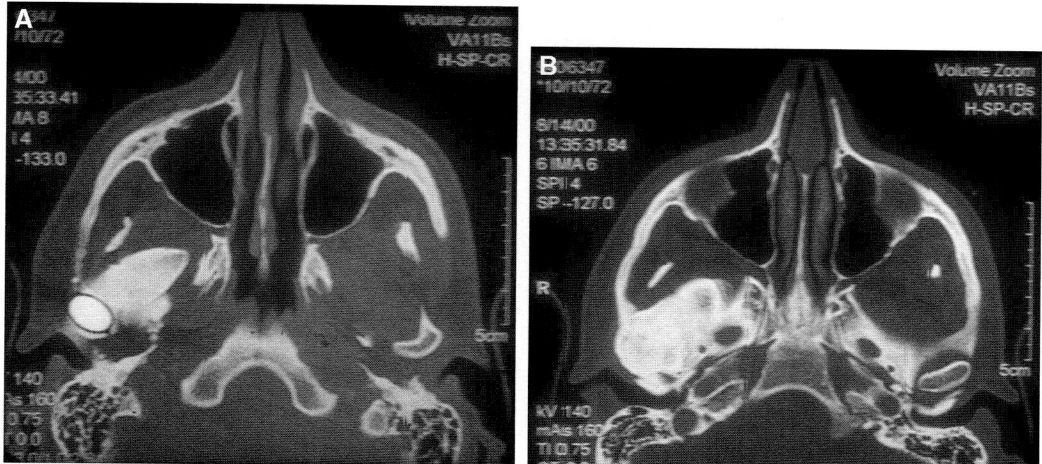

Fig. 2. Axial CT scans of the same patient in Fig. 1. (*A*) at the level of the condyles, (*B*) bone ankylosis at the base of the skull surrounding the condylar prosthesis is seen.

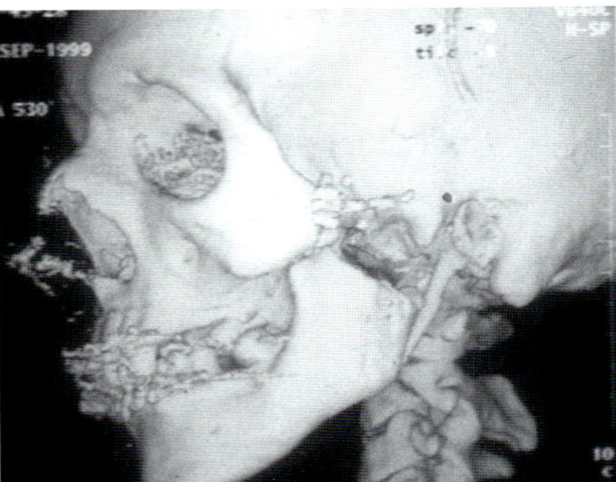

Fig. 3. Three-dimensional CT scan of another patient after mandibular mobilization surgery. Note that the ankylotic mass has been excised from the skull base down to the level of the mandibular lingula.

Preparation for the total joint

The glenoid fossa must be shaped to receive the fossa prosthesis. Irregular bone should be smoothed and a shallow fossa created. The fossa should be as horizontal as possible, because lateral forces tend to dislodge the prosthesis over time. The lateral aspect of the arch should be inspected and prepared for the flange of the prosthesis. The lateral surface of the mandible should be prepared to receive the condylar prosthesis. Excess bone, old costochondral grafts, and hardware should be removed. Areas in which foreign body reaction has destroyed bone should be débrided thoroughly. In these cases, the prosthesis may need to extend onto the body of the mandible.

Temporary prosthesis

A temporary condylar prosthesis is used to maintain occlusion and restore function. Abdominal fat can be packed around the prosthesis in the dead space created by the excision

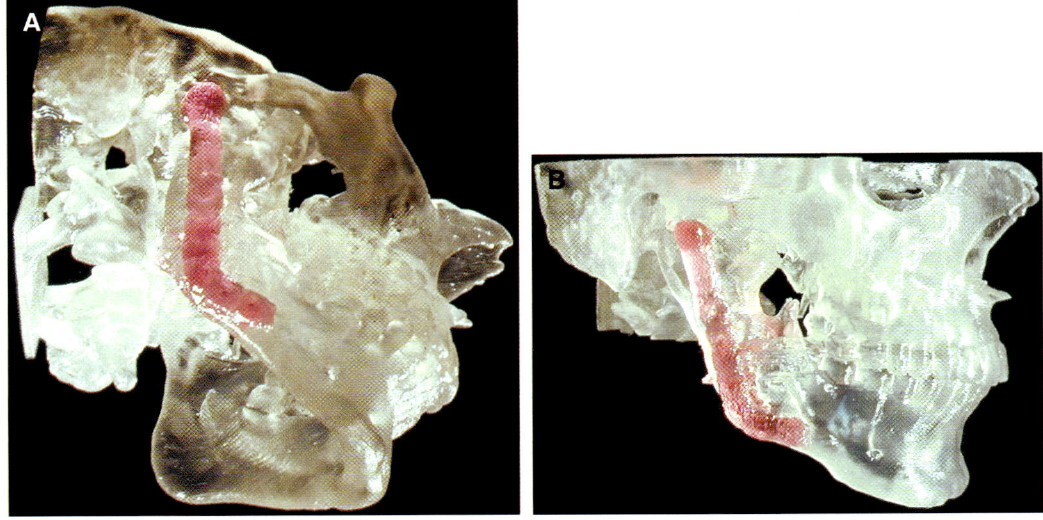

Fig. 4. Stereolithographic models made for the patient in Figs. 1 and 2. (*A*) Oblique view. (*B*) Lateral view. Note the reconstructive plate in red. It is surrounded on the medial and anterior aspect by bone. The styloid process is elongated and fused to the posterior border of the mandible.

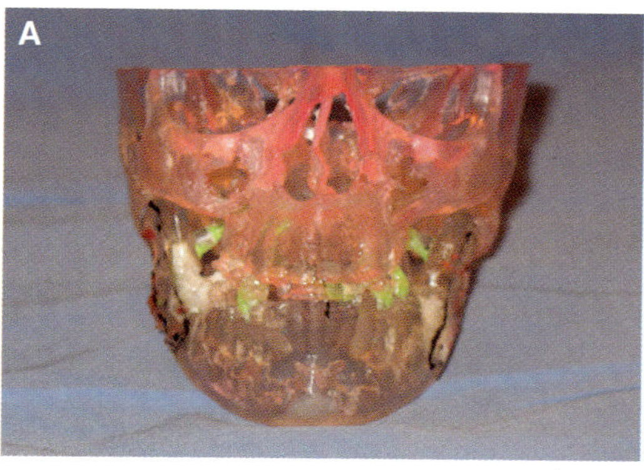

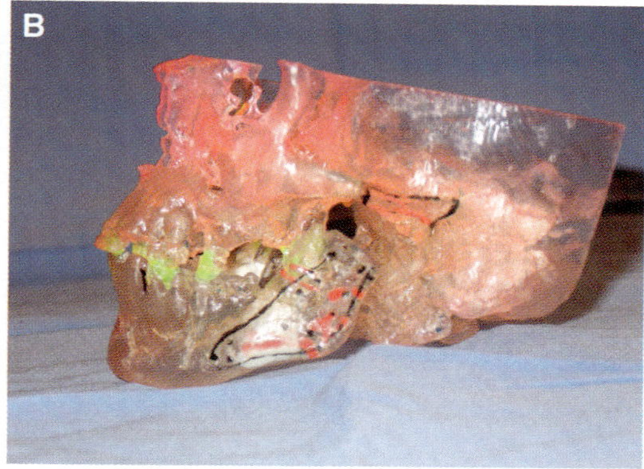

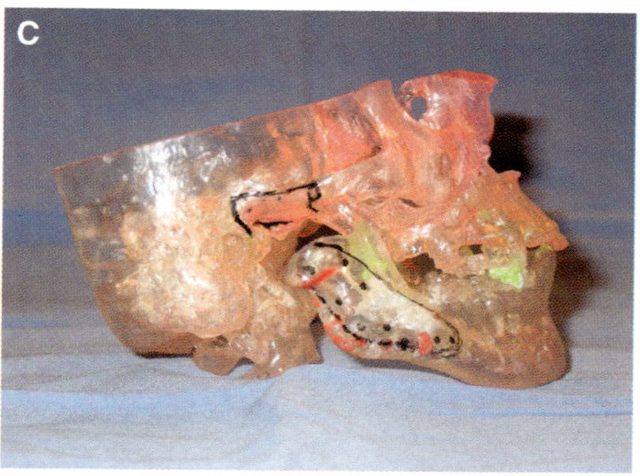

Fig. 5. Stereolithographic models made for a different patient. The model is prepared with the coronoid removed to the lingula. The prosthesis is outlined, and the screw placement is marked out. (*A*) Frontal; (*B*) Left; (*C*) Right.

of the ankylotic mass to prevent scar tissue formation. After surgery, a second three-dimensional CT scan is taken and a stereolithographic model is constructed.

Evaluation of stereolithographic model

Once the stereolithographic model (Fig. 4) is made, the surgeon must inspect it to ensure that a sufficient gap has been created between the base of skull and ramus. The surgeon also must confirm that sufficient coronoid process has been removed, bilaterally, if necessary. Finally, the glenoid fossa and lateral surface of ramus are confirmed to be smooth and prepared for the construction of the prosthesis. The model is then trimmed until the desired anatomy is achieved. A written record of these changes should be kept and the areas carefully marked out on the model (Figs. 5 and 6).

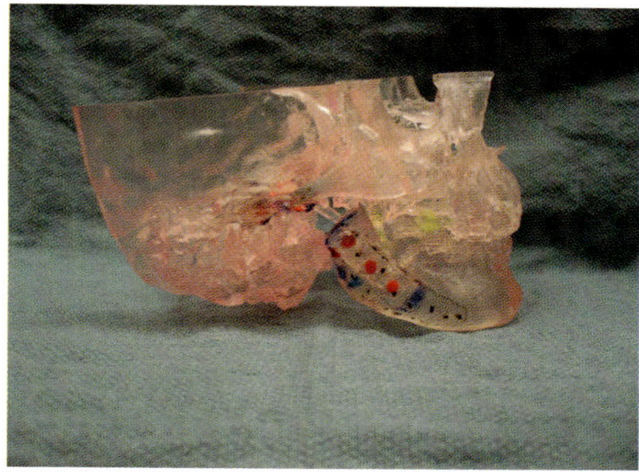

Fig. 6. Stereolithographic model made for another patient. Note how the prosthesis will be extended onto the body of the mandible to be stabilized to healthy bone.

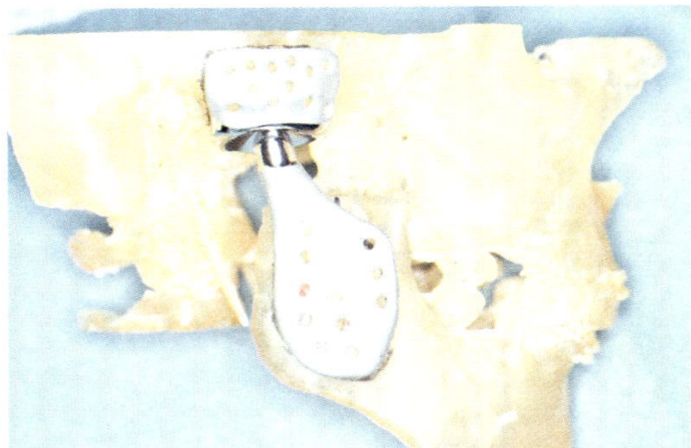

Fig. 7. Photograph of the custom-made prosthesis (TMJ Implants Inc, Golden, CO) on the model. The fit of the prosthesis is confirmed. This is the prosthesis for the patient in Figs. 1, 2, and 4.

The manufacturer creates wax templates. On these templates the surgeon must ensure that the glenoid fossa prosthesis covers the involved area at the base of the skull and that the articulating surface is horizontal. The placement of screw holes also should be verified (Fig. 5). The surgeon should ensure that the screw holes for the condylar prosthesis avoid the inferior alveolar nerve canal. Finally, the angulation of the condyle must be checked. If the condyle is too obliquely angled, it should be extended posterior to the angle to provide a more vertical angulation with the glenoid fossa. The prosthesis may need to extend onto the body of the mandible to stabilize it in sound bone (Fig. 6). The wax template with any adjustments can be returned to the manufacturer for the construction of the custom-made prosthesis (Fig. 7).

Second-stage surgery

During the second-stage surgery, the temporary condylar prosthesis is removed. The adjustments made to the stereolithographic model are reproduced in the bone. The range of

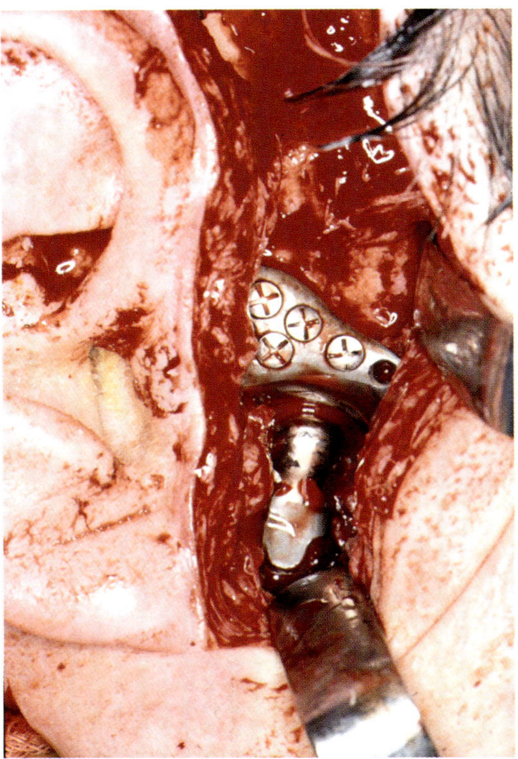

Fig. 8. Intraoperative photograph of the same patient in Figs. 1, 2, 4, and 7, with the total joint prosthesis in place.

motion is checked to ensure that adequate mobilization has been achieved. The custom-made fossa is fitted, and any fibro-osseous tissue in the area is removed thoroughly to achieve full and stable seating of the prosthesis. This process is crucial, because a poorly fitting prosthesis eventually loosens. A template with holes is provided to help the surgeon at this stage. The glenoid fossa prosthesis is screwed into place. The condylar prosthesis is fitted, and any changes made to the stereolithographic model are reproduced. Any fibro-osseous tissue is removed thoroughly to ensure that the prosthesis is stable and completely seated (Fig. 8). The occlusion is checked. The fit and motion of the condylar prosthesis in the fossa prosthesis are verified.

Further readings

Mercuri LG, Wolford LM, Sanders B, et al. Long-term follow-up of the CAD/CAM patient fitted total temporomandibular joint reconstruction system. J Oral Maxillofac Surg 2002;60(12):1440–8.

Wolford LM. Temporomandibular joint devices: treatment factors and outcomes. Oral Surg Oral Med Oral Pathol Oral Radiol Endod 1997;83(1):143–9.

Wolford LM, Dingwerth DJ, Talwar RM, et al. Comparison of 2 temporomandibular joint total joint prosthesis systems. J Oral Maxillofac Surg 2003;61(6):685–90; discussion 690.

Wolford LM, Pitta MC, Reiche-Fischel O, et al. TMJ concepts/Techmedica custom-made TMJ total joint prosthesis: 5-year follow-up study. Int J Oral Maxillofac Surg 2003;32(3):268–74.

Changing Your Address?

Make sure your subscription changes too! When you notify us of your new address, you can help make our job easier by including an exact copy of your Clinics label number with your old address (see illustration below.) This number identifies you to our computer system and will speed the processing of your address change. Please be sure this label number accompanies your old address and your corrected address—you can send an old Clinics label with your number on it or just copy it exactly and send it to the address listed below.

We appreciate your help in our attempt to give you continuous coverage. Thank you.

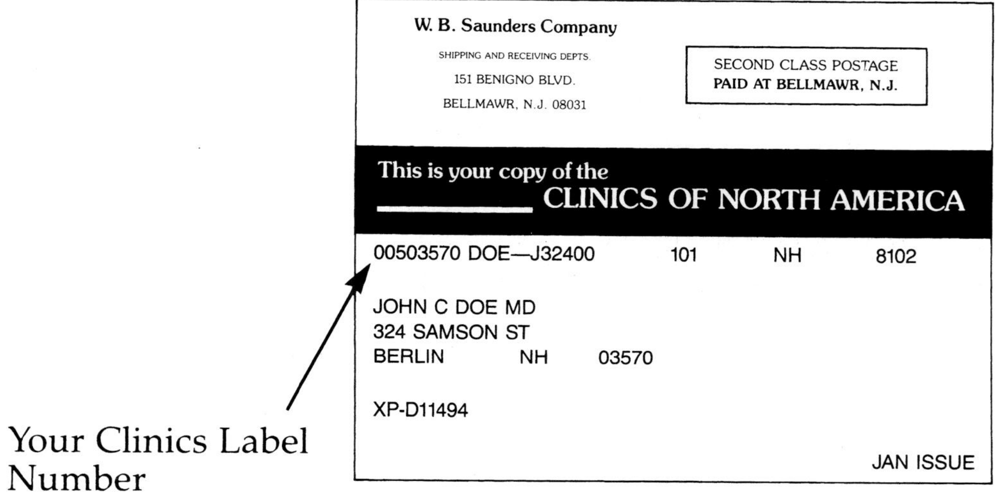

Copy it exactly or send your label along with your address to:
W.B. Saunders Company, Customer Service
Orlando, FL 32887-4800
Call Toll Free 1-800-654-2452

Please allow four to six weeks for delivery of new subscriptions and for processing address changes.